C000062482

Tall Life

Sam Lochner PhD

© 2016 Sam Lochner

Illustrations by Taras Kharechko

Cover by Sumit Roy

All Rights Reserved

No part of this publication may be reproduced, stored in a retrieval system, or transmitted, in any form or by any means, electronic, mechanical, photocopying, recording, or otherwise, without the written permission of the author.

Please do not participate in or encourage piracy of copyrighted materials in violation of the author's rights. Purchase only authorized editions.

First published by Sam Lochner

Kitchener, Ontario, Canada

www.Tall.Life

ISBN: 978-0-9952102-1-9

Table of Contents

AUDIENCE

While I have written this book primarily to benefit tall people, the intended audience is much broader than just tall people. For instance, medical and exercise professionals who have tall clients will find this book informative and helpful in their practices. Something similar can be said for designers, regulators, teachers, researchers, and even family and friends. Additionally, anyone with an interest in height in general or the covered topics will find this book fascinating.

INTRODUCTION

For the same reason that things are rarely manufactured for tall people, there aren't many books written for us either; it's not economical given how few of us there are. This doesn't mean there aren't important things to say—quite the contrary. In fact, there's a massive void in the literature on tall stature. I hope this book will begin to fill it.

If you search the web, you'll find out some great things about being tall—like the fact that we tend to have more successful careers. But you'll hear a whole lot more about the problems. Giving weight to this is the popularity of the phrase, "tall people problems". The phrase "tall people solutions", on the other hand, is virtually unheard of. So this book is fairly unique in that the purpose is to solve the problems. It's also to raise awareness and give perspective. Along the way, I'm certain you'll also learn some fascinating, even astonishing things about your height.

At 6'7", I've been compared to a giraffe on more than one occasion. The giraffe-tall person comparison has become a cliché. However, besides both being relatively tall, there's a lot more to this comparison than most people are aware of. And surprisingly, it's actually our differences with giraffes that can reveal the most important implications of tall stature. After you read the first chapter, Evolution, I think you'll agree that nothing could be more appropriate than a giraffe for the cover of this book.

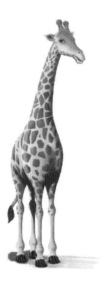

In the second chapter, Scaling, I explain how the properties of the body change with height. For instance, while we have greater absolute strength, we actually have lesser relative strength, as per the square-cube law. This explains why we're good at lifting heavy things but then struggle with push-ups and chin-ups. Similarly, while we use more energy in the absolute sense, we actually use less in the relative sense.

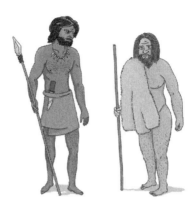

In the third chapter, Spine, I discuss our increased risk of injuries, particularly back injuries. The usual explanations are "longer levers" and "The bigger they are, the harder they fall". But aren't our bigger bodies also stronger? And if large size is such a problem, then how is it that giraffes get by? I answer these questions in this chapter. I also present some practical suggestions on exercises, activities, and strategies to prevent and recover from back injuries, all in the context of tall stature. Much of this chapter draws on the work of the world renowned spine researcher, Stuart McGill, whom I had the good fortune of meeting while struggling with my own back pain.

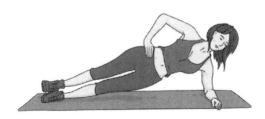

While we're naturally at greater risk of injury, the ergonomic hazards caused by ill-fitting manufactured objects, like cars, desks, and kitchens, worsen matters. As to why these hazards exist, that's because of a mechanism known as the economy of scale. But such advancements as mass customization, on-demand manufacturing, and 3D printing will make life easier for us. All this is covered in chapter four, Manufactured, along with my own personal case study on cars.

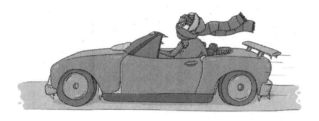

The full realization of these advancements may not occur for some time. While we wait, we can learn to better adapt. This is the topic of the fifth chapter, Ergonomics. Being a DIY enthusiast, I've had a lot of fun with adapting. I've made a long snow shovel, a raised cutting board, and some handy modifications to my methodically selected car. More generally, I've adapted how I interact with most objects. I share all of this in this most practical chapter.

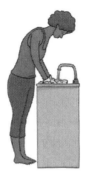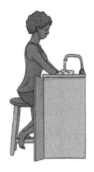

For the remainder of the book, I transition away from the mechanical perspective. In the sixth chapter, Growth, I briefly summarize how people grow tall in the first place and how to predict adult height. I also summarize height-related disorders, recognize some of the world's tallest people, and explore the bizarre business of intentionally shrinking people.

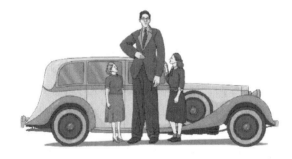

I'd never actually heard of this practice until I started researching for this book. Perhaps this is because society associates tall stature with many benefits including good health. However, recently there's mounting evidence that extremely tall people, such as myself, are at increased risk of disease. The data on cancer risk is particularly convincing. The common explanation is that tall people have more cells and so a higher probability of developing cancer. But if size is such a problem, then how can it be that larger species tend to live longer? I answer this question and more in chapter seven, Longevity, while touching on perspective and prevention.

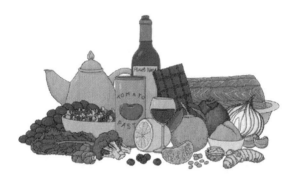

Unlike the topics I've mentioned thus far, the social issues revolving around tall stature get a fair bit of media coverage. Specifically, the fact that we tend to earn more money and have more successful careers draws a lot of envy, to the point where a 'tall tax' has been proposed. Similarly, there are those wishing to weed us out of the human race because of our supposed greater usage of the planet's resources. And parallel to all this, society crams us into tiny cars and airplane seats. I tackle all of these issues in chapter eight, Society. Also in this chapter are some positive and helpful insights for tall women.

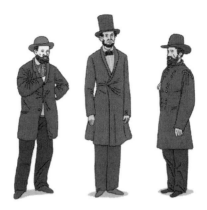

Finally, the Afterward is my own tall tale of the events that led to the writing of this book. In particular, I go into detail about the role my height played in becoming a chronic back pain sufferer, but also how I recovered.

I've ordered the chapters of this book so as to first build a theoretical foundation before moving on to the more practical content. However, I've also written them in such a way that they can stand on their own. So, please consider beginning with whatever chapter interests you most. Think of this book as a kind of resource to be referred back to rather than a story you read from start to finish only once.

Before getting started, let's consider the title of this book. The first word is a rather popular one. If you search the web for the word 'tall', you get over half a billion results at the time of writing this. But what does it mean?

In the broadest sense, tall simply means above average height. A more technical definition is, two standard deviations above average. This is about the ninety-eighth percentile. To help distinguish between various degrees of tall, I like to use the terms 'kinda tall' and 'extremely tall' as shown in the curves below that I created from US height data.[1] These curves would of course change for different populations and ages.

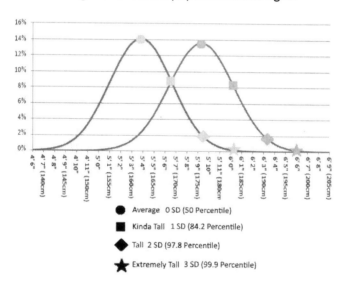

● Average   0 SD (50 Percentile)

■ Kinda Tall   1 SD (84.2 Percentile)

◆ Tall   2 SD (97.8 Percentile)

★ Extremely Tall   3 SD (99.9 Percentile)

From these curves, it's clear that most people are near average, some are kinda tall, few are tall, and extremely tall people are rare indeed. Being an outlier has considerable implications both in the artificial and natural sense. Throughout this book, I show that being tall affects just about every aspect of our lives.

And this is why 'life' is the second word in the title of this book. It's an even more popular word, with nearly six billion search results. This is perhaps because of its broad usage. It can be used anywhere from the pop culture sense as in a lifestyle magazine, to the most scientific as in the existence and workings of an organism. As you'll see, it's applicable in this book across the spectrum.

When you take these two words of the title, Tall and Life, and put a dot between them, you get the address of the website that carries on the discussion of height and tall stature beyond the covers or bytes of this book. As you work your way through this book, please check out www.Tall.Life and join in the discussion.

Finally, I'd like mention a few points on my own expertise. I have a PhD in mechanical engineering and my research and work have related to mass customization and biomechanics. This expertise is only relevant for about half the book. Nevertheless, given my experience as a researcher, I'm confident that I've done a decent job on the rest of the book. Really though, I don't intend for this book to be for anything other than information purposes. For more than that, I'd point you to the many books and journal articles I cite and professionals I mention.

Now, without further ado, let's turn to our tall friends, the giraffes, as we cultivate an understanding of human height and tall stature through the lens of evolutionary theory.

EVOLUTION

"... man with all his noble qualities... still bears in his bodily frame the indelible stamp of his lowly origin."

—Charles Darwin

Evolutionary forces affect human height. Hence, these forces must be considered if a discussion on tall stature is to be complete. Giraffes make for excellent examples for such a discussion, given they, like tall people, are recognized for their exceptional vertical extent. What may surprise you though, is that it's actually how we're different from giraffes that's most telling.

This chapter and the next one build a theoretical foundation. So it was logical to place them at the beginning of the book. However, many readers will prefer to start elsewhere, perhaps with Ergonomics, the most practical chapter, or Society, the most widely relatable chapter. As I mentioned in the introduction, I wrote the chapters such that they can be read in any order.

The Evolution of Height

I find that if I stand up too quickly, I get a head rush and sometimes even start to black out a bit. I don't know if I'd ever actually fall over because of this, but I've learned to grab something solid just in case. I used to think that this was normal, that it happened to everyone just as much. It wasn't until I started studying engineering that I realized that my being tall makes me more liable for this.

A taller column of blood has a greater pressure differential, and this is amplified when quickly rising. The result is a greater blood pressure drop in the brain. This is called orthostatic or postural hypotension and studies confirm the fact that tall people are more likely to experience it.[2,3] There can be many side effects, including dizziness and a temporary loss of vision.

All this got me wondering about how giraffes get by, given their towering necks. For instance, imagine a giraffe is busying drinking water with its head way down low. Then suddenly it senses a lion and quickly raises its head. Why wouldn't a pressure drop result, causing it to pass out and provide a tasty snack for the lion?

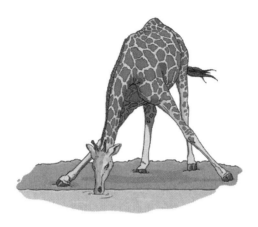

The explanation is that giraffes have special adaptations to deal with their enormous height. They have valves in their jugular veins to prevent blood from flowing back down to the head when lowered,[4] and then other mechanisms to assist in bringing blood up to the head when raised.[5] They acquired these adaptations through the process of evolution. Let me briefly introduce this process by summarizing Darwin's explanation for giraffe's exceptional height.

Just like with people, young giraffes tend to grow up to be a lot like their parents, though with some small differences. For instance, some giraffes just happen to end up a bit taller than their parents. And while giraffes in general are great at reaching leaves way up in tree tops, taller giraffes are even better. This is particularly important in times of scarcity and can actually make the difference between life and death. And when taller giraffes survive, they get the chance to reproduce and have tall calves of their own. In this way, height can gradually increase as generations pass. Over millions of years, Darwin explained, this evolutionary process known as natural selection led to giraffes extraordinary stature.

Humans, of course, don't need to be tall for grazing purposes. But there are other potential advantages of increased height. I'll explain some of these in more detail in the next chapter. To summarize though, taller humans have better reach, visibility, speed, absolute strength, heat retention, and energy efficiency. But there are also advantages to shorter stature including maneuverability, agility, relative strength, heat dissipation, and lesser energy requirements.

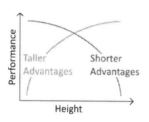 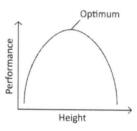

When you combine these performance trade-offs in a given environment and plot them versus height, you get an inverted U-shaped curve. The peak of this curve corresponds with optimum height for that environment. As an environment changes, so will the optimum height. Natural selection will then cause population height to follow suit.

For example, consider that most pivotal point when our ape-like ancestors finally left the comfort of their trees.[6] As to why they left, it probably wasn't because they got bored of swinging around like a bunch of monkeys. Rather, it was more likely enforced by an environmental transition from mostly forest to mostly open plains. And once down on the ground, it was advantageous to be taller; this meant greater ability to see predators, and also speed to escape them. The taller of our ancestors were then fortunate enough to stick around and have potentially taller kids of their own. Population height could have trended upwards in this way.

But there are also factors that would work to decrease stature, like insufficient food for our voracious appetites. In the long run though, it's clear that height has trended upwards. We're not alone in this trend towards increasing size. What is referred to as Cope's rule states that all lineages tend to increase in body size over time.[7]

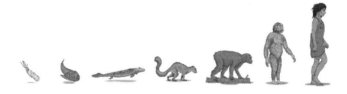

Yet this increasing in size occurs most gradually, in small increments. Giraffes, for example, have taken millions of years to reach their current height. This has afforded them, via natural selection, ample opportunity to adapt for this height. This is in stark contrast to tall people given we've most likely reached our additional size above our species' average in a mere few generations. This is why we, unlike giraffes, are prone to head rushes.

But a bit of blacking out is the least of our concerns, particularly because we tend to keep nearby lions caged up. Far more problematic is our increased risk of musculoskeletal injuries, arrhythmias, and cancer, as well as our lesser reproductive success. I talk about these issues in the chapters to come.

A useful analogy here is the design of buildings. Over time, architects have gradually learned how to design taller buildings as they gained knowledge from past experiences. If an eighteenth century architect, on the other hand, had just up and decided to out of the blue build the Burj Khalifa, which at least for now is the world's tallest building, it surely would have been a disaster. Of course this is the extreme case, but much like for tall humans, it holds that unusually tall buildings miss out on the same extent of optimization as buildings of more common heights.

People often wonder about how we'll evolve in the future, whether or not we'll continue to grow taller. As I noted above, the general trend in nature is gradually upwards. Yet the laws of scaling do eventually begin to apply downward pressure, as I explain in the next chapter. Beyond even this though, mass extinctions tend to be less kind to the largest species, the dinosaurs being the classic example. This is known as the Lilliput Effect. Environmental changes that could cause mass extinctions include famines, epidemics, natural disasters, asteroid collisions, and climate change perhaps from global warming or cooling.

Some have actually suggested that we should intentionally shrink the human race to reduce our environmental toll and decrease the risk of famines. But there are counter arguments to this I present in the final chapter. One point I make is that there are other more crucial cultural and technological advancement to thwart such disasters. In the event these are sufficient, perhaps we'll in fact continue to grow taller, as per Cope's rule.

CHAPTER 2

SCALING

"...the ratio of two volumes is greater than the ratio of their surfaces"

—Galileo

Tall people tend to be stronger. This is well known. Less well known though is that, relative to our own weight, we actually tend to be weaker. This explains how we can be good at lifting heavy things, but then struggle with push-ups and chin-ups. In this chapter, I explain this and other size related characteristics with the laws of scaling.

This chapter expands on the theoretical foundation from the last chapter. After this chapter, the remainder of the book will be more practical.

Proportional

The word proportional is a rather common one. It's used a lot in the context of human height and shape. For example, perhaps you've heard a friend say something along the lines of, "She is proportional." What they might have meant is that the ratio of her leg length to her torso length is what it ought to be. Similarly, her head and feet may look to be the right size for her body, and so on.

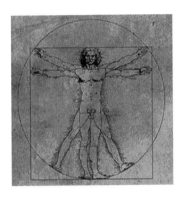

With "ought to be" and "right size", an ideal set of proportions is implied. Leonardo Da Vinci also presented this same implication with his Vitruvian Man. No overall dimensions were specified, but rather only relative dimensions. For instance, he wrote that the body is eight heads tall. In other words, the height of the head is proportional to the height of the body.

To explore proportionality of the human body further, a box can be a useful analogy. Assume length (L) and width (W) are both proportional to height (H). If the height of the box is doubled while maintaining this proportionality, then both length and width must also double as in the illustration below.

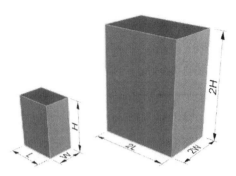

This is an over simplification of how people scale. Yet this approximation, in combination with the square-cube law, is helpful when explaining why and how the properties of the body change with height.

The Square-Cube Law

The words tall and short refer to the vertical extent of something. So we call a person with a greater vertical extent tall, and lesser short. But this can be misleading, as there are much greater differences than merely vertical extent between short and tall people. In fact, the fundamental properties of the body vary with height. The square-cube law can explain why.

Take a look at our smaller box from the previous section. As I already mentioned, doubling its height while maintaining proportions results in length and width also doubling. Less obvious though is that volume increases more than area, twice as much to be exact. This is because three-dimensional volume is proportional to the cube of height while two-dimensional area is merely proportional to the square of height. Galileo might have been the first to formally recognize this when he stated in his 1638 book, *Two New Sciences*, "...the ratio of two volumes is greater than the ratio of their surfaces."

This is enormously important as so much depends on the ratio of volume to area. For example, weight is proportional to volume while strength is proportional to area. So while strength increases with size, in relation to weight it actually decreases. Another way to say this is that the larger body is **absolutely** stronger but **relatively** weaker.

The classic example of this is a comparison between an elephant and an ant. The elephant is stronger, this is most obvious. Where the ant excels, though, is in being able to carry a great many times its own body weight. You see this when ants are carrying food many times their own size back to their queen. Elephants clearly can't do this. The elephant is absolutely stronger but the ant is relatively stronger. This trend with size is present not just for ants and elephants, but all animals, even humans.

So while tall people have greater absolute strength, we have lesser relative strength. This is why tall people, like world record holding 6'6" Behdad Salimi Kordasiabi, can lift more weight but then aren't as good at push-ups and chin-ups.[8] Coaches, drill-sergeants, and the like really need to be alerted to this fact. The square-cube law can also explain why tall people, like 6'5" Usaine Bolt, may be lightning fast yet make for poor gymnasts due to a lesser ability to accelerate body mass.

Lower relative strength also translates to higher stress, the force per unit of area. You can think of stress like pressure, which we use to measure the inflation of tires, often with units of pounds per square inch. Stress, rather than simply force, is what counts when it comes to musculoskeletal injuries. I talk about this more in the next chapter.

Beyond the mechanical, the square-cube law has implications for many other aspects of the body, such as thermal properties. Heat generated and contained is a function of volume while heat dissipated is a function of surface area. This means that we should bear cold weather better but then be more likely to overheat in hot weather or during exertion. More on this later though.

This heat transfer relationship also means that our taller bodies lose relatively less energy to the external environment, which in turn coincides with a lower metabolic rate in relation to mass. In other words, our bodies are less energy efficient in the absolute sense, yet more so in the relative sense. This will prove most consequential in chapter seven, Longevity.

In this section we've assumed that proportions are maintained as people scale, that tall people are just enlarged versions of average people. This approximation is helpful for explaining how and why the body's properties change with size. But it's just that, an approximation. The point of the next section is to consider how people actually scale.

Scaling Variations

In case you haven't heard of the Body Mass Index (BMI), it's basically an equation for evaluating the healthiness of your weight for your height. Underweight people get a low number, overweight a high number.

Given I'm a rather slim guy (6'7" and 215 lbs), I was totally shocked when the BMI labelled me as overweight. I did a little digging and it turns out I'm not alone here—this is typical for tall people in general.

Where the BMI goes astray is that it assumes people scale with the square of height, meaning they get a whole lot thinner as they get taller. Tall people do tend to be thinner,[9] but only moderately. By exaggerating how thin we are, even the healthy among us are labeled as overweight. This is a major issue given the BMI is used for important purposes including determining insurance premiums. Plus it's just plain annoying.

This inspired me to build a calculator for what I like to call the Better Body Mass Index. It's based on the fact that people scale somewhere between height squared and height cubed.[10–12] You can find the calculator on www.Tall.Life. Despite how it better accounts for variations in height, it still shares the BMI's limitations of not accounting for muscle mass, ethnicity, nor gender.

Let's focus in on the main point of this section, which is that tall people tend to be **moderately** thinner. This does of course make for different properties than if proportions were maintained. However, the relationships I explained in the previous section are merely diminished. For example, we still tend to be absolutely stronger but relatively weaker. Similarly, we should fare better in a cold climate but worse in a warm climate.

However, this relationship swaps when a particularly slim build is combined with exceptionally long limbs, as relative surface area actually increases. For example, our long limbed and slender Cro-Magnon ancestors would have fared better in a warm climate than barrel chested Neanderthals, despite being taller.

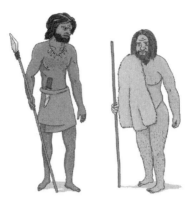

Besides variations in overall proportions, more subtle variations occur throughout the body. For example, while we have bigger heads, these tend to be smaller in relation to the rest of our body. In parallel to this, we have bigger brains, but not proportionally bigger. Nevertheless, bigger brains tend to be better, and this has been used as one possible explanation for the height-intelligence positive correlation.[13,14]

Bone mass tends to go the opposite direction, meaning we become relatively more big-boned. This is necessary, as per the square-cube law, to support greater body mass. To highlight this point, let's proportionally scale our aforementioned ant up to the elephant's size. Note how tiny the ant's legs look in comparison to the elephant's. Clearly this mutant ant's legs would collapse under its own weight. Unlike the mutant ant, the elephant has achieved its great mass over millions of years, providing it ample opportunity to adapt to thwart injury. Large members of species, such as ourselves,

25

may not adapt as effectively—more on this in the next chapter.

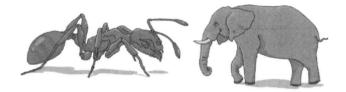

Finally, I'd like to note that biological variations can only go so far and the laws of physics eventually do start to cap species' size. As size increases, ability to run is eventually lost, which is eventually followed by the loss of ability to support body weight. For instance, the largest dinosaurs did not run and Godzilla could never exist on Earth. To get a most profound appreciation of the far reaching limitations that the laws of physics impose on size, consider that there's a cap on the maximum size of a rocky planet that won't collapse in on itself. Low density gas planets, on the other hand, can be much larger.

SPINE

"The bigger they are, the harder they fall."

—5'1" Barbados Joe Walcott, Former World Welterweight Boxing
Champion

Taller people are at increased risk of injury. In this
chapter, I explain why this is the case, focusing in on
back injuries in particular. I also discuss some exercises,
activities, and spine sparing strategies that can help in
the prevention and recovery from back injuries.

Much of this chapter draws on the work of the world
renowned spine researcher, Stuart McGill, whom I had
the good fortune of meeting while I was struggling with
back pain of my own. If you want to learn from the
expert himself, I suggest starting with his latest book,
Back Mechanic.[15]

Height and Back Injuries

Barbados Joe Walcott, the 5'1" former world
welterweight boxing champion, was well known for

entering into matches against significantly larger opponents. His rather famous reasoning was that, "The bigger they are, the harder they fall," and he figured a smaller fighter could take advantage of this. For anyone other than Barbados Joe Walcott, this would probably be a bad bet. But, he was right that a larger person experiences more force when they hit the ground.

But shouldn't our taller bodies be better suited to larger forces? They are, but not proportionally so. This is because the taller body, despite being absolutely stronger, is relatively weaker. I explained this in the previous chapter via the square-cube law.

Another issue often pointed out is that our larger bodies have longer levers. To better appreciate this concept, let's consider the wrench analogy. As we all know, it's hard to get a nut off a bolt by hand. This is why we have wrenches. And for the tightest nuts, we have extra-long wrenches. This is because a longer wrench can apply more torque (rotational force) to the nut. But while large torque is great for unscrewing a nut, too much can break it. Similarly, taller people's longer limbs apply more torque to the joints. And as with forces, our larger joints are better at accepting larger torques, but not proportionally so, as per the square-cube law. The result is an increased risk of injury.

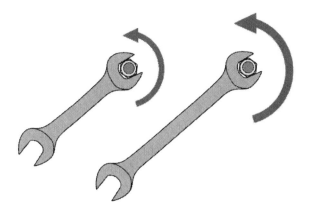

Another issue tall people face is that a thicker body experiences more stress when bent or twisted a given angle. You can verify this yourself by bending two different size wooden dowels, noting that the thicker one breaks at a lesser angle.

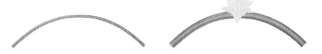

And yet one more issue is our slower reflexes that result from longer nerves,[16–18] as this makes it harder to avoid injurious situations. All of these issues, and perhaps more, increase our risk of injury.

But if size is such an issue, then how is it that larger species get by? Shouldn't giraffes be constantly suffering from sore necks? The answer is that larger species have had millions of years to adapt for their great size, such as by becoming relatively more big boned. Their legs also tend to be stacked closer to vertical, including when running, and this decreases torques on their joints.[19] More generally, they move conservatively and plan far ahead in order to compensate for their slower reflexes.[20] Tall people have not benefited from this same extent of evolutionary adaptation for our size, and this, rather than our size alone, is the deeper reason why we're more likely to become injured.

Many studies confirm that we're at greater risk for injuries, including to the ankle, knee, hip, back, neck, shoulder, and wrist.[21–34] Studies of injury rates in various sports also routinely find tall athletes are at greater risk.[22,31–33] And the injuries that afflict the elderly are also more common in tall people, such as hip fractures.[34]

I've injured all but one of the joints I mentioned above. My worst injury by far was to my back. Back injuries can come on suddenly, or gradually as was the case for me. I figure poor posture has a lot to do with it, or more specifically, a deviation from neutral spine posture. This is more likely to occur for tall people both due to ill-fitting manufactured objects and lesser relative strength. But what is it that's so disastrous about deviating from neutral spine posture in the first place?

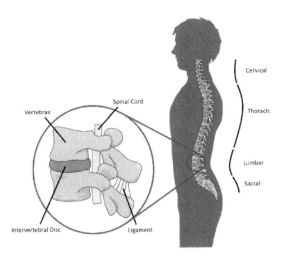

A deviation from neutral spine posture corresponds with a bending of the spine. The main problem with a bent spine, Stuart McGill explains, is that uneven pressure is applied to the discs.[35] This is particularly problematic for loads that are large (car accident), applied over longer durations (desk work), or applied cyclically (vibrating machinery or sports). Uneven pressure in these instances pushes the gel-like contents of the disc away from center, encouraging a departure from the disc. The simplest way to visualize this is as the squishing of a jelly donut. Sometimes the result is called a herniated disc. I have several discs in my own spine that have been damaged similarly.

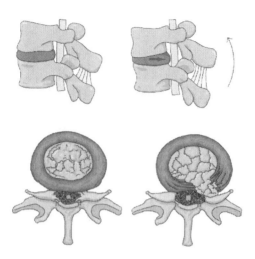

Another way discs can become altered is by a loss of water content, which results in a decrease in thickness. This happens naturally over the course of the day as gravity compresses the discs. This is why we tend to be shorter in the evening than in the morning. I actually once bought a car in the evening only to find out the next morning that it was too small for me!

As we age, the discs can lose some of their ability to remain hydrated, and this results in a more permanent reduction in stature. Besides with age though, desiccation can also result from stress, which in theory tall people are more subject too. Once again, many of my discs have been damaged in this way.

As I know from experience, disc damage can cause immense pain. This may come directly from the damaged disc or from the pressure herniations put on sensitive nerves outside the disc. Pain in turn causes tightness, putting more stress on the discs. The resulting injury loop can lead to chronic pain.

Though there's some evidence that discs can regenerate,[36,37] this healing is nowhere near as speedy as for broken bones. One doctor actually told me mine would probably never heal. The fact I wish he'd have told me, though, is that herniated discs and the like are often asymptomatic,[38] meaning there are lots of people walking around with them without even knowing it. It would follow then that herniations may become asymptomatic with time. Knowing this early on would have saved me a lot of grief.

To give the discs a chance to become asymptomatic, we must avoid injuring them further. So in this case, prevention and recovery are pretty much the same thing. The key for both is maintaining good posture. This can be aided by modifying ill-fitting manufactured objects and how we interact with them. I give some examples for how to do this in chapter five, Ergonomics. Beyond this, there are some exercises, activities, and spine sparing strategies that can help, and these are the focus of the remainder of this chapter.

Spine Stabilizing Exercises

When my back first started getting bad, I jumped to the conclusion that this was a sign of weakness. So I hit the gym and started lifting some heavy weights. Similarly, I was told I had to improve my flexibility, so I began working my way up to being able to touch my toes with straight legs, and so on.

As it turns out, I was doing myself more harm than good; I later learned from Stuart McGill that neither high static back strength nor mobility are associated with lower risk of back injury, and can actually have the opposite effect. Instead, it's good muscle endurance and control that's important. For further appreciation of this notion, consider that low force tasks extended over long durations, such as standing, or tasks requiring proficient control, such as picking a pencil up off the ground, often lead to injury.

Muscle endurance and control are thus important for maintaining a stable spine, where a given posture, usually the neutral posture, is maintained. This ability can be improved with exercises that challenge endurance and control, such as *Stuart McGill's Big Three Stabilizing Exercises.*[35] I briefly explain these below. Before attempting these, it's best to consult a physiotherapist or similar.

Cat-Camel: This first exercise isn't for increasing stability but rather for increasing the viscosity in the spine, among other benefits, and thus useful for preparing for stabilizing exercises. McGill recommends moving between these two postures approximately five to eight times, integrating movement throughout the entire spine.

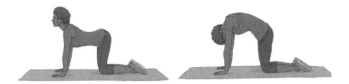

#1 Curl-up: With the hands supporting the neutral curvature of the low back and one knee flexed, the head and shoulders are slightly raised from the floor. A possible routine could include three sets with six, four, and then two reps that last ten seconds each, alternating which knee is flexed.

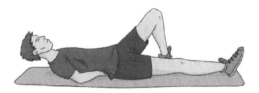

#2 Side Bridge: Support the body weight by the feet and forearm. The less advanced version is done with the knees on the ground. The same rep/set pattern as for the curl-up can be used.

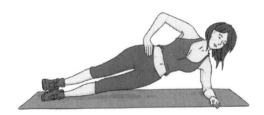

#3 Bird Dog: One arm and one leg, on opposite sides of the body, are raised. The same rep/set pattern as the curl-up can be used.

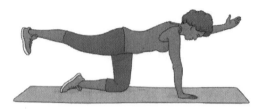

Posture Correcting Exercises

A former coach of mine once mentioned to me that I looked strong from in front but weak from behind. What he was noticing was that my chest muscles were overpowering my upper back muscles, causing my shoulders to round forward.

Some years later, I learned that what I was experiencing was part of a fairly common pattern of muscle imbalances known as the crossed syndromes.[39,40] They're called crossed because tight and weak compensations literally cross the body, cascading along its length in an alternating pattern. In the spine, visually, the tight regions are curved inwards while the weak and elongated regions are curved outwards, both contributing to an accentuation of the spine's natural curvatures.

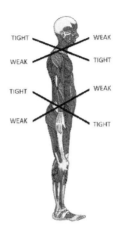

There are two characteristics of the crossed syndromes that warrant pointing out in the context of tall stature. The first is that the resulting distorted posture relies more on passive support from musculoskeletal tissues, thereby decreasing muscular effort. The second is that they decrease overall stature. Taller peoples' diminished relative strength and relatively short artificial environment may provide increased incentive for us to adopt the distorted posture, and thereby initiate the syndromes.

Besides the crossed syndromes, there are many other ways posture can become distorted. The good news though is that regularly performed exercises can provide some compensation for the issues leading to postural distortions. The basic idea is to stretch the tight muscles and strengthen the weakened muscles. A physiotherapist or similar can help determine if your posture is distorted and prescribe exercises to correct it.

Activities

When my back first got bad, I got a lot of suggestions for various activities I could do that might help. Perhaps the most common was to do yoga, for which the benefits for back pain sufferers are well known.[41,42]

Many yoga poses help build muscle endurance and control and correct common postural distortions. Particularly beneficial are the poses that emphasize neutral spine posture. And beyond the mechanical aspects, there are other reasons why yoga may be helpful for back pain sufferers, including the cultivation of mindfulness.[43,44]

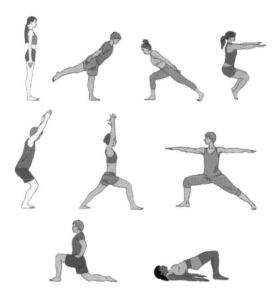

I'd like to note, though, that Stuart McGill has expressed concern over the yoga poses that twist and bend the spine considerably, such as those below. He explains that this isn't necessary for building a robust back, and can actually increase the risk of injury. Yet, as McGill demonstrated in a recent yoga workshop I attended, some of these poses can be done more moderately or modified for the individual, which happens to be a central theme in yoga.

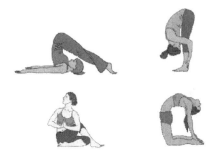

I think yoga is particularly great for tall people given it presents an opportunity to improve relative strength, which we tend to lack. The flip side though is that we need to be careful with the poses that require high relative strength. Our other characteristics that warrant caution include lesser flexibility, more numerous injuries, and thicker spine that won't twist nor bend as readily. Nevertheless, I've been practicing yoga with moderation myself for some seven years now and am certain that it has helped me enormously.

The next most common recommendation I got was to take up swimming. This seemed like a great idea to me, particularly because tall people, like 6'4" Michael

Phelps, make great swimmers. As with yoga though, swimming is a varied activity, so different strokes for different folks. The Phelps style butterfly, for example, will probably not be helpful to those suffering from back injuries. Breast stroke and front crawl, on the other hand, may be better. But even these require some extent of twisting and extending of the spine as breaths are taken. The solution I came across is to use a swim snorkel. This negates coming up for air, thereby facilitating a neutral posture along the entire length of the spine.

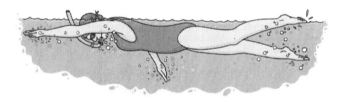

When swimming is vigorous, it yields cardiovascular benefits, which can be beneficial for back pain sufferers.[45] This is likely because of a hypoalgesic effect[46]; endorphins are released which decrease pain much like morphine does. Extended exercise can also trigger the release of endocannabinoids which can give a euphoric feeling commonly known as runner's high,[47] helping the body to relax. I've found cycling to be an even better form of low impact cardiovascular exercise. McGill does point out though that competitive road cycling can encourage too much spine flexion.

Walking, though somewhat less than cycling and swimming, also has cardiovascular benefits. Interestingly, McGill has found a brisk pace—and for tall people this will be particularly fast—better for the back than a stroll. A decent arm swing and looking straight ahead also help. More walking can be interjected into daily life by parking at the far side of the lot, taking the stairs, and my personal favorite, getting a dog.

Food can also have an influence on injury recovery and prevention, including on the body's inflammation response. Sufficient consumption of Omega-3s in particular has been recognized as important.[48]

A final concept I'd like to mention is moderation. A routine, whether for an athlete of any level or for an individual recovering from an injury, lies on an inverted U-shaped curve, where the optimum has neither too much rest nor too much training.[35] By finding this golden mean, as Aristotle once called it, optimum physique can be achieved.

Spine Sparing Strategies

Young people, my former self included, tend not to be all that careful with their backs. For instance, I remember my total disregard for spine posture when lifting things, despite my wiser elders advising me to keep a straight back. I did eventually learn, but the hard way, and at great cost to my spine. Perhaps if I'd read it in a book such as this, it might have played out differently. Below are a variety of spine sparing strategies.

- **Maintain a neutral spine posture:** Neutral spine posture is particularly important when under load, especially prolonged static and cyclical loads.
- **Use the lower extremities for getting low:** The squat, hip hinge, lunge, and golfer's lift are all robust postures for getting low.

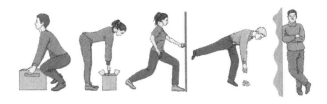

- **Minimize torque arms:** By lifting close to the body and pushing and pulling through the center of the spine, torque acting on the spine is minimized. When pulling low door handles, for example, torque can be reduced via a slight lunge.
- **Contract core muscles before lifting heavy loads:** Though this increases the load on the spine, it ensures the neutral posture is maintained, which tends to be more critical.
- **Use aids:** Use lifting tools such as hoists, dollies, and furniture straps. Protective clothing can also help as it encourages holding the load closer to the body, thereby reducing torques.

Knee pads are particularly helpful for us as they encourage getting low via kneeling rather than flexing the spine.

- **Use mechanical advantage:** When lifting a log, for example, use leverage by lifting one side at a time. Better yet, have a second person lift the other side as is common in such tasks as moving a couch.

- **Avoid prolonged static postures:** Even low stresses, when maintained for long periods such as for desk work, can lead to injury. So it's best to regularly get up and move.

- **Avoid bending and lifting early in the morning and after sitting:** The discs are most hydrated after waking, and this leads to a stiff spine. Sitting tends to have the opposite effect, but only on one side of the spine. It's best to delay bending and strenuous activity after both waking and sitting.

Another factor that needs addressing is the poor ergonomics that result from ill-fitting objects. I get to the root of this problem in the next chapter, followed by possibilities for adaption in chapter five, Ergonomics.

CHAPTER 4

MANUFACTURED

"... the creation of a new power, namely, the collective power of masses."

—Karl Marx

One of the challenges of being tall is that manufactured things rarely fit us. This is true for clothes, airplane seats, and just about anything manufactured. As much as this might feel like some sort of conspiracy, it isn't. In this chapter, I explain the real source for this bewildering predicament once and for all. I also get into how grading of sizes and building in adjustability helps, as well as the ultimate solutions, on-demand manufacturing and mass customization.

I conclude the chapter with my own case study on cars, the most hazardous of manufactured objects for us.

The Economy of Scale
I like to buy most of my food at the local farmers' market. One of many benefits is that it tends to be

cheaper. This is particularly true when I buy apples by the bushel. I'm sure you've appreciated something like this at some point too. But have you ever actually thought about why it's cheaper to buy in quantity?

Consider that the price of each apple is the sum of the costs from growing it right up until you purchase it. Some of these costs will be variable, meaning they're directly proportional to the number of apples sold. An example is water to grow the apples. Water tends to be sold at a set price per a given volume no matter how much you use, within reason. You can see this on your water bill. If all costs were similarly variable, then the cost per apple would be independent of quantity.

However, there are also fixed costs. For example, land is required to grow the apples, a truck is required to drive the apples to the market, a booth is required to sell the apples, and employees must run the show. When these fixed costs are divided over a larger number of apples, the price per apple decreases. Furthermore, larger fixed costs are relatively cheaper. For instance, a larger plot of land will be cheaper per acre and something similar can be said for the truck and the booth.

Sometimes the laws of scaling come into play, specifically the square-cube law. Consider living accommodations. We all want single detached homes, but these can be pricey. A duplex is slightly cheaper for many reasons. One is heating costs are lower given the shared wall that isn't exposed to the elements. Apartments are even better in this regard. In general, the larger the building the better as relative surface area decreases with size. Besides heating costs, there are many other scaling based sources for savings from construction materials to utility networks.

The point I'm trying to make thus far is that greater quantity yields lower prices. This mechanism is commonly known as the economy of scale. It's because of this mechanism that larger quantities of apples are cheaper per apple, a benefit that's passed down to the consumer who buys in larger quantities. Economies of scale such as these are what has led to production in ever greater volume by ever larger entities, as was foreseen by the German philosopher, Karl Marx.[49]

By now you may be wondering what this has to do with tall people in the first place. If you remember back to the curve in the introduction, it showed that there are far fewer people in the tall-range than the mid-range. And because of this, as a group, we're purchasing in smaller quantities. These quantities are akin to the basket rather than bushel of apples, and so we must pay more.

But often we aren't willing to pay more. Hence, companies simply neglect us and instead focus on the masses. This results in inconveniences, like ill-fitting clothing.

Worse though, yet still due to this same lack of economy, ergonomic hazards occur, as seen in work environments and transportation. Not even medical devices, as alarming as this may be, are exempt from this predicament. And beyond objects, human knowledge also revolves around the average height person.

Entrepreneurs, tall ones in particular, are constantly recognizing the need for tall specific clothing and other products. However, some may not realize that it isn't because few have perceived it that this need exists. Rather, it's because this need is expensive to address. Nevertheless, there are niche companies out there that are geared towards tall consumers. These of course are typically online businesses, avoiding the fixed costs of a brick-and-mortar location. Other aspects of a business that suffer from a lack of scale do still present challenges. These include software licenses, liability insurance, any outsourced work, and building rent.

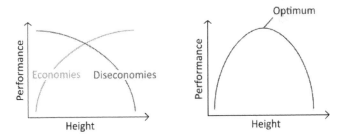

Economy does not increase indefinitely with volume of goods produced. Similar to how evolutionary forces lead to optimal animal size, there are also factors that lead to optimal operation size. In the example of the apple business, bottlenecks in the supply chain, such as a shortage of workers or pesticides, will actually decrease economy with scale. This is known as diseconomy of scale, and when combined with economy of scale, forms an inverted U-shaped curve. Unfortunately for us, the peak of this curve tends to coincide with far greater quantities than we require.

However, there's another phenomenon that can become a factor, and that's disruptive technologies and paradigm shifts. These can have a sudden impact on an industry. Two such advancements that will be helpful to tall people are mass customization and on-demand manufacturing, which I touch on later.

Next up are the currently practiced approaches of grading of sizes and building in adjustability.

Grading and Adjustability

There are a couple of ways manufacturers are able to feasibly cater to a broad range of sizes. The first is by simply grading a standard size up rather than developing an entirely new design. The second is by building adjustability into products. However, both of these approaches have shortcomings.

Let's consider clothing for an example of multiple sizes, beginning with shirts. The basic shirt sizes are small, medium, and large. This single dimension of variation means that the lengths and girths are tied together. Hence if someone is tall **and** thin, not only will they have trouble finding a shirt long enough, it will inevitably be overly baggy. This is worsened by clothes shortening but widening with washing and drying.[50] Likewise, the truly big **and** tall will find shirts to be both too short and too narrow. And while the smallest of people have the option of wearing children's clothing, no such repurposing exists for us.

However, it must be conceded that the situation has improved somewhat in recent years as more brands begin to offer a range of sizes in tall form, more big and tall stores pop up (technically they're big **or** tall stores), and some niche companies cater specifically to very tall people.

Pants are somewhat better than shirts, typically varying by both length and width, as in a two-dimensional array of sizes. This creates a band rather than line of possible body shapes that can be accommodated. High-end footwear does similarly. Providing a third dimension would further improve matters. Yet the number of sizes that must be stocked is increasing exponentially with each additional dimension. The cost of designing, manufacturing, shipping, and stocking the resulting number of sizes isn't practical, thereby limiting the usefulness of this approach.

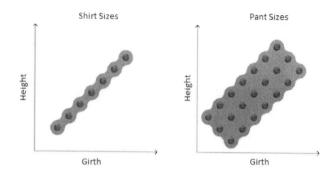

Shirt Sizes   Pant Sizes

And then there are situations where providing multiple sizes isn't practical. Consider airplane seats, for example. Within a given class, any individual may occupy any seat, so multiple sizes isn't an option. Instead, airlines attempt to provide some degree of accommodation via adjustability, specifically by allowing seat backs to recline. But given airplane seats' notoriety for discomfort, this degree of adjustment is clearly inadequate. Legroom in particular, which reclining detracts from, is a problem and I come back to it in chapter eight, Society.

Just like with increasing number of sizes, increasing number of adjustments improves the level of accommodation. The basic car seat that both tilts and slides will be better than the airplane seat, and the high-end office chair with half a dozen adjustments will be even better. However, even these high-end office chairs will often not accommodate the tallest of people.

The products that accommodate the greatest range in body size and shape, as noted by Arianne Cohen,[51] tend to be those that offer both multiple sizes **and** adjustability. The bicycle is a fine example. Simply by providing seat and handlebar adjustments, designers have been able to accommodate the geometry of a high percentage of the population with around ten sizes.

Regardless of the approach used, accommodating all different body sizes and shapes is a costly endeavor. So companies must compromise by deciding on a reasonable level of accommodation. The low end limits the number of customers who find the product suitable while the high-end carries a prohibitive cost. Once again, we see the inverted U-shaped curve, where there's an optimal level of accommodation to maximize profit.

Depending on the scenario, the level of accommodation for maximal profit may be rather low, thereby encouraging the design of products that could be unsafe. In these instances, governmental regulators should step in.

The automobile, which I arrive at in a couple sections from now, makes for an interesting example to explore these issues more deeply. Next up though is the manufacturing trends that may diminish the need for grading and adjustability as they shape another industrial revolution.

The Next Industrial Revolution

Once upon a time, clothing and other articles were made one at a time, and specifically for the wearer. This was a time consuming and expensive endeavor, and many would often have to do without.

The first industrial revolution changed all this. New manufacturing methods were adopted that made it possible to produce textiles and other goods in large quantities, thereby harnessing the economies of scale and making these goods affordable for the masses. The problem that arose, though, was that the resulting articles only fit near-average size individuals.

The digital revolution came somewhat later. The resulting computer-aided technologies improved mass production methods, but also presented a new possibility; by simply changing the computer code, products differentiated for the individual could be made.

This presents considerable opportunity in the footwear industry in particular. I should know about this given I've been involved in the development of custom footwear technology for some years now. What I've come to realize is that there's still a long way to go. In fact, a pair of truly custom shoes still costs in the thousands of dollars. You heard me right, thousands! The problem is that there remain too many fixed costs.

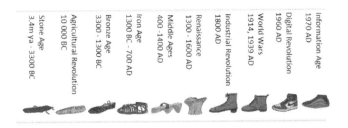

Information Age
1970 AD

Digital Revolution
1960 AD

World Wars
1914, 1939 AD

Industrial Revolution
1800 AD

Renaissance
1300 - 1600 AD

Middle Ages
400 - 1400 AD

Iron Age
1300 BC - 700 AD

Bronze Age
3300 - 1300 BC

Agricultural Revolution
10 000 BC

Stone Age
3.4m ya - 3300 BC

However, a new manufacturing approach referred to as additive manufacturing, which includes 3D printing, has enormous potential. Unlike subtractive manufacturing, material isn't cut away, but rather added up. This reduces waste while permitting for both more complex geometry and multiple materials.

When additive manufacturing methods reach maturity, it will be possible to produce both a greater variety of products on-demand, thereby more easily catering to outlier populations, and products specifically designed for the individual, as in mass customization. The latter is aided by the development of 3D scanners which are used to create a 3D model of the body about which products can be designed.

However, a switch to predominantly variable costs introduces a new problem. Consider that a pair of shoes currently costs the same for all sizes, despite how the larger sizes require more material. This is because pricing models reflect cost structure, which are mostly fixed. But as costs become mostly variable, the pricing models will follow suit. For 3D printing, for example, pricing models are mostly based on geometric volume which is related to the cost of raw material and machine time, with just a small setup fee. And given tall people require footwear and other articles with larger geometric volume, we'll pay more.

Nevertheless, this next industrial revolution will remove many of the obstacles for companies wishing to include or even cater to outliers such as ourselves. There's a total disruption of the manufacturing industry on its way, and we'll benefit, and the entrepreneurs among us should be jumping on the bandwagon.

To complete this chapter, the next section is a kind of personal case study on cars, the most hazardous of manufactured objects for us.

Cars

Cars have played an important role in my life. I started driving at the youngest age possible. This was encouraged by my separated parents given they would no longer have to drive a combined eight hours each weekend to trade me off. My first car was a 1986 Toyota Corolla, twelve years old at the time. It cost just eight hundred bucks and I could watch the road fly by through a hole in the rusted out floor. But it got me from A to B.

The car only lasted me about a year. Over the next decade, I found myself driving a new old car every year. A lot, but when you have a DIY car guy like my father was, I'm guessing this is par for the course. These cars varied from a tough old Ford 150 pickup truck to a family friendly minivan. But what they all had in common was that I didn't fit. Though of course I wasn't fully aware of just how hunched I must have been until some years later when I sat in my tiny Corolla once more (my father had a way of keeping things around until they became one with the earth once more). All this got me wondering why cars are so poorly suited to us.

As with other manufactured objects, economy of scale encourages manufacturers to cater to average height and neglect outliers. There are regulations that help. But these tend to be inadequate for tall people. For example, common regulations merely require accommodation of the fifth percentile female through to the ninety-fifth percentile male,[52] leaving five percent of the population unaccommodated. In actuality, this percentage is higher due to varying body proportions.

This low level of accommodation leads to a major health hazard for us. A lack of legroom can affect reaction time for hitting the brakes,[53] increasing the likelihood of an accident. And if an accident does occur, more serious injuries are likely to result; airbags, low head rests, and insufficient legroom have all been implicated in more serious injuries experienced by us in a crash.[54–56] Even outside the car our safety is relatively diminished; bumpers are designed to cause minimum damage when striking average length legs, not long legs.[57] These are some of the more obvious implications. Somewhat less obvious is the gradual insidious onset of chronic musculoskeletal injuries that arise from poor ergonomics.

It didn't dawn on me that a low head rest was such a problem until my Toyota 4Runner was hit from behind by a distracted driver watching a peanut shaped hot air balloon (she actually conceded this to the police officer). Lucky for me, it was a low speed collision, and I escaped with just a neck ache. But I can understand how a low headrest in a more serious collision would increase our risk of whiplash injury. It's totally inexcusable that car companies don't add that couple extra inches to the head rest rails to save us this. What would it cost, a few cents?

Similarly, why can't we have a few extra inches of seat rail so we can move our seats further back? Even if we could though, the fore-aft adjustment is somewhat flawed in the first place. This is because humans have longer legs than arms, so moving the seat back far enough for the legs will move it too far for the arms. Another issue is that a longer torso, even at a slight seat angle, puts the shoulder joints even further from the steering wheel. The consequence of these issues is that we often find ourselves hunching to reach the steering wheel, despite how we have such long arms.

Exacerbating matters is the fact that we tend to recline our seats to gain headroom, forcing us to hunch even more. After my 4Runner got written off, I remember testing out a purple Elantra. It was a fun little car, but I didn't fit. The sales guy tried to convince me to tilt my seat back and 'relax'. Had I headed his advice, my spine would be far worse off today. Plus I'd be driving a purple car.

A somewhat less common adjustment is seat height. When it comes to chairs other than car seats, we obviously prefer taller ones. When it comes to cars, though, we'll choose to **lower** our seat in order to gain headroom. In fact, I've actually tried removing seat foam to get even lower. But I've found this to be a poor compensation as a lower seat compromises legroom, flexing the hip, knee, and ankle joints too much.

I'm looking forward to someday getting a high-end car given they typically have some additional adjustments that can help in dealing with some of these issues. Telescoping steering wheels and pedals can compensate for the legroom/reach discrepancy while tilting seat pans can better support the thighs. There are also adjustable lumbar supports, seat belts with adjustable shoulder height, etc. Though these adjustments are certainly helpful, the range of adjustment could be better. And frustratingly, these higher end models tend to come with headroom-stealing sunroofs. And no, it does not make sense to ride with your head out the sunroof! Similarly, a convertible isn't the answer either.

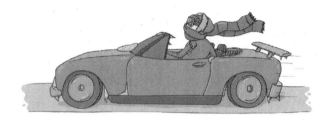

The level of adjustability required to make us comfortable in a standard car is simply impractical. Hence, multiple sizes are required. Yet not even a single production car, despite there being thousands of models out there, is geared specifically towards us. This seems astoundingly unfair when you look at the lavish advancements currently being made, from parallel parking automation to sophisticated entertainment and communication systems. Perhaps the regulations that have helped us are hindering in this instance, as any car must suit the fifth percentile female. Or perhaps the research just doesn't show that the market size is feasible, given the strong economy of scale in car production. Regardless, we're on our own to sift through existing cars in hopes of finding one that a designer inadvertently made suitable.

I talked to a lot of people when I first started looking for a more suitable car. The common advice I got was to get a big truck. This idea is a glaring misconception; overall size poorly correlates with cabin height. Though the Humvee may look tall, this is due to ground clearance rather than cabin height. Ironically, a Mini Cooper is more comfortable for the tall driver than many large SUVs and pickup trucks.

Next, I turned to the manufacturer's websites, looking up the various measurements. These were helpful, though I should mention they're somewhat inconsistent; interpretations of the *Society of Automotive Engineers'* (SAE) standard measurements vary. The two most useful specified measurements for us are legroom and headroom.

Legroom is a measure of the longest leg that can fit in the seat while in its most aft position. The measurement is complicated by the bending of the knee joint. Though the standards require that a dummy be used to take the measurement, a good approximation can be achieved via a tape measure.

Headroom is the vertical distance, with the seat in the lowest position, from the lowest point on the seat to a point on the roof directly above it. I've found headroom to be a misleading measurement as cars differ in the extent to which the roof rises above the vision line; though it may be comfortable to occupy this space, it's dangerous to do so as visibility is cut off. So an alternative measurement would instead go to the top of the windshield. I like to call this 'eyeroom'.

Another measurement I have come up with is called Vision Line Height (VLH). It's the vertical distance from the foot well (floor mat removed) to where the windshield meets the roof. VLH is a measurement of **useful** cabin space, essentially.

Both eyeroom and VLH are better than headroom for picking out the top cars for tall people. As to which is better, this is debatable. For those willing to do modifications, VLH will be better. Otherwise, eyeroom might be better. But VLH has the added bonuses of being simple to measure and also evaluating how easy a car is to get into and out of; even small increases in roof height have been shown to improve posture during ingress and egress.[58] When I was searching for my own car, I was desperate to find something that permitted me a straight spine, even if that meant seat modifications, so I went with VLH.

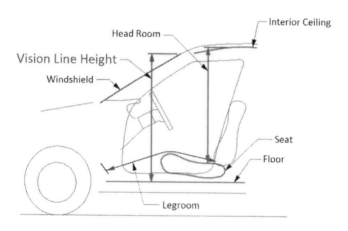

Armed with my newly coined VLH measurement, I hit the dealerships, measuring every car they had. This was much to the bemusement of the sales people who just wanted to make a sale. To keep them motivated, I said I'd buy any car they sat me in where my head didn't touch the roof. Needless to say, I made them no richer... until I came across the Honda Element.

With a VLH of 46-⅝", one of the best out there, it's no surprise that the Honda Element is often talked about on tall forums. Besides being tall friendly, I think it's arguably the most versatile car to be made in recent years. Infuriatingly, it was discontinued in 2011.

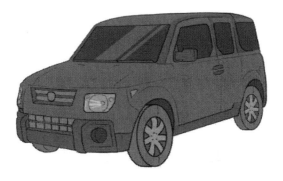

Another top tall car, the Scion XB, was redesigned as of 2007 to be shorter and then finally discontinued in 2015. Similar to how human height is a variation in the human genome that can either be naturally selected or not, variation in car height is also a variation of sorts within the automotive industry that can be artificially selected or not. In this case, not. For the Honda Element, perhaps it was a sexual selection of sorts, as many have proclaimed it ugly. Form appears to have won out over function.

Take reassurance, however, in that a new champion has arrived in town, and that's the Ford Transit Connect consumer model with a whopping 51-½" VLH. Its roots were as a small and efficient in-town delivery vehicle where a high windshield allowed delivery people to see high-up building numbers and signs. Its popularity promoted it to consumer vehicle status around 2011. Here's hoping they neither discontinue it, nor drop the roof anytime soon.

An even more promising solution lingers on the horizon, and that's 3D printed cars. The Urbee, perhaps the first of its kind, uses a 3D printed body. Further down the road it will be possible to 3D print even more of the car. Suddenly, variations in car geometry become cheaper as costly jigs and molds are no longer required. It may be possible, someday down the road, for cars to be made in multiple sizes and perhaps even tailored to the driver.

However, there's a growing sentiment that our current usage of cars is unsustainable. This is because of pollution, inaccessibility for people who don't drive, and impaired drivers. Perhaps the most likely replacement will revolve around electric robotized smaller forms of public transportation that can go door to door. The troubling word here is smaller; if these things are designed for the masses, and thus cater to the average size, it will be a chore for us to stand up for more space. Hopefully, knock on wood while there still is some, these things won't go down the same dark path as airplane seats.

But while we await the pros and cons of future cars, we must cope with the challenges presented by today's automobiles along with the many other unsuitable objects of human origin. This can be done by adapting our ergonomics, which is the focus of the next chapter.

CHAPTER 5

ERGONOMICS

"Adapt or perish, now as ever, is nature's inexorable imperative."

—H. G. Wells

In the previous chapter, I shed some light on why manufacturers neglect us, but also how a new paradigm will improve matters. In the meantime, however, ill-fitting manufactured objects create ergonomic hazards that amplify our already greater risk of injury. The solution is to adapt our ergonomics, which is the focus of this chapter.

I begin the chapter with a short but formal introduction to the field of ergonomics. After that, we'll get to the fun stuff.

Ergonomics and its Principles

We are constantly interacting with our physical environment. There's a variety of approaches we can take to carry out any given interaction. Yet there exists an approach that yields an optimal combination of performance and wellbeing. Ergonomics, or in this case, physical ergonomics, is the study which aims to find such an approach.

I've compiled the following list of basic ergonomic principles from a variety of sources, including the *Centers for Disease Control's National Institute for Occupational Health and Safety*. Note that these points overlap with those in the spine sparing strategies list in chapter three, Spine, where I provided more detail.

- Reduce force and torque (rotational force)
- Alternate postures
- Keep everything in easy reach
- Work at proper heights
- Reduce excessive motion
- Minimize fatigue and static load
- Minimize pressure points
- Ensure sufficient clearance
- Move, exercise, and stretch
- Maintain comfortable environment
- Maintain neutral joint position

Many of these recommendations are more difficult for tall people to follow. For example, low work surfaces and cramped cars encourage poor posture which can gradually lead to spinal degeneration, ill-fitting seats cause pressure points which can lead to clots, and low objects are sources for head injuries. These issues may also diminish efficiency. However, by adapting, we can circumvent many of these issues. In the next section, I present some tall solutions for a variety of situations.

Tall Solutions

At last, we've made it to my favorite part of this book, the stuff that inspired me to write it in the first place. As to why I like these tall solutions so much, well they helped me escape from years of chronic back pain. Also, I simply enjoy the DIY approach, which is usually the only feasible option for us so neglected tall folk.

The tall solutions I cover in this section fall under two categories. The first is where the object being interacted with is adapted. The key principle here is that the interaction between the tall person and the adapted object should be similar to that of the average person and the original object. For example, if the work surface was intended for average elbow height, then the adapted work surface should be at the taller person's elbow height. The same is true for joint angles; an adapted computer workstation should allow for similar joint angles for the tall person as does a standard workstation for the average person.

Adapting the object may not always be possible, which brings me to the second type of tall solution. With this, we change how we interact with the object to circumvent the ergonomic issue. For example, when avoiding low hanging objects, we should flex the ankles, hips, and knees rather than the spine, thereby preserving the spine.

We can apply these two approaches to adapting to a great variety of situations. In some cases, adaptations may be somewhere between the two. In the following sections, I describe solutions for some specific situations. Please note that I've covered some of these in more detail on www.Tall.Life.

Tool Handles

Whether you're mowing the lawn, pushing a stroller, or pulling your luggage, chances are you're doing it at a far less than ideal height. Handles just aren't designed for us. Even the adjustable ones tend to have inadequate range. The solution is to extend the handles. In some cases, there are existing handle extensions you can purchase such as those for wheelchairs, lawnmowers, strollers, and luggage.

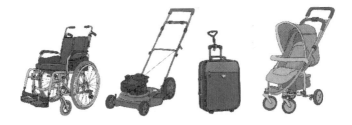

Once again though, these may not be long enough. In this case, it's often possible to build an extension yourself. My favorite example is the snow shovel, partly because shoveling snow is notorious for causing back injuries even for average height people. One way to adapt a snow shovel handle is by removing the existing shaft and replacing it with a longer one. I've done this with a wooden dowel from the hardware store. Most snow shovels come up to around the shoulder for the average height person, and so the adapted snow shovel should do the same for the taller person. Other tools such as brooms, rakes, and spades can be adapted similarly.

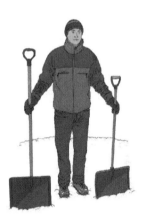

Kitchen

Kitchen work is an ergonomic nightmare for us as, in addition to static postures, reaching, and repetitive tasks, surface heights are too low. Kitchen surfaces are typically three feet high, which is intended for the average height female (5'4") doing the average kitchen task. So kitchen counters are too low for more than half the population, and way too low for us.

I have a couple friends that have had their kitchens built with higher surfaces. But they've generally had to compromise on the height given they live with shorter people and also because they don't want to affect resale value. The ultimate solution is adjustable surface heights. However, this is a fairly pricey investment and you likely won't get your money back if you sell.

The alternative I've come up with is to use a raised cutting board. There are many ways to build one. The basic idea is to attach legs to a regular cutting board. The same could be done for a wooden countertop. What's great about this solution is that you can make it any height you want, move it when it's not needed, and it's super cheap. It helps to do the cutting on a secondary cutting board as this is then easier to clean. Another quick tip is to keep a compost bin beneath the cutting board that can be pulled out to catch scraps.

Whether building a custom kitchen or simply raising a cutting board, you must decide upon a suitable height. One to two inches below elbow height has been found comfortable for most kitchen tasks (finer tasks require higher surfaces and vice versa).[59] This translates to a 6'7" person, such as myself, using a one foot rise, approximately. This may seem extreme at first, but only because we're accustomed to working at improper heights. One helpful approach to arriving at a satisfactory height is to stack books beneath a cutting board, gradually increasing the height.

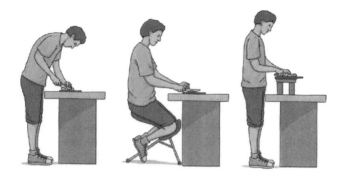

When raising isn't an option, we should instead lower ourselves. I used to do this with a kind of semi-splits, and this got a lot of laughs. The more comfortable solution I've come up with is to pair a seat with a surface that yields a good relative work surface height. With the many varieties of seats (chairs, kneeling chairs, and stools) and surfaces (dining room table, kitchen counters, and island), there's sure to be a suitable combination. For doing work at the sink, I've found that a stool works particularly well while opening the cupboard doors to provide space for the knees. I've heard this can be made more convenient by installing a hanging, swinging stool (like you see in pubs) and cupboard door hinges that open up beyond ninety degrees.

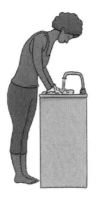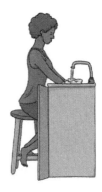

Besides work surfaces, other objects in the kitchen also require getting low. These include cupboards, drawers, dishwashers, and fridges (freezer drawer on bottom style is better). Rather than slouching through the spine, this is best done by using the ankles, hips, and knees as in lunging, squatting, kneeling, and hip hinging. If you have hard floors that hurt your knees, keep a towel or foam pad handy. I sometimes don my old volleyball kneepads when I've got a lot of housework or a repair job to do.

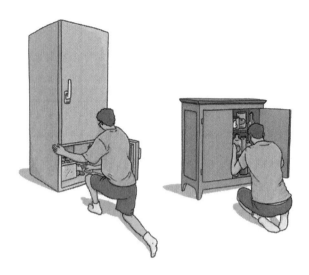

While a standard kitchen may at first appear to be a hindrance, with some adaptation it can actually be preferable. For example, while I like to use a raised surface for chopping vegetables, I actually prefer to use the lower surfaces for other tasks such as kneading dough or unloading groceries. Similarly, sink bottoms are too low for even average height people, but with a stool the tall person can achieve superior ergonomics.

Dining Room

In addition to ergonomic issues, etiquette also presents challenges for us in the dining room. In particular, we're supposed to sit up straight with our elbows off the table, making for an awkwardly large plate to mouth chasm. And the communal nature of the dining room makes it challenging for us to adapt.

When my back was really bad, I was so desperate to keep a straight spine that I used to use a couple rather quirky solutions. The first was to find myself a lower chair, and sit in a semi-cross-legged position. The second was to use what I call a raised placement, which is a shorter version of a raised cutting board essentially.

A more permanent solution I've come up with involves a pub style table and chair set. The idea is that average height people sit as was intended, with their feet resting on a chair rung, kind of like they're in an adult sized high chair. We, on the other hand, can either adapt a pub chair or use a standard or custom chair.

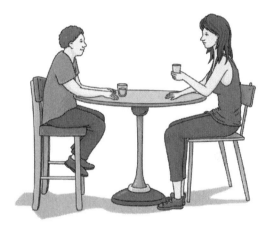

Desk Work

As we spend more time working with computers, workstation ergonomics becomes ever more important. There's a variety of schools of thought on how computer workstations should be set up. As an

example, below are some points proposed by the
*United States Department of Labor's Occupational
Safety and Health Administration* as well as computer
monitor position recommendations by the *Canadian
Centre for Occupational Health and Safety*.

- Hands, wrists, and forearms are straight, in-line, and roughly parallel to the floor
- Head is level or tilted slightly downwards, forward facing, and balanced. Generally it is in-line with the torso
- The monitor should be positioned between sixteen and twenty-eight inches from the face and such that the center of the monitor is slightly below fifteen degrees from horizontal. Make sure the top of the monitor is not above eye level
- Shoulders are relaxed and upper arms hang normally at the side of the body
- Elbows stay in close to the body and are bent between ninety and one hundred twenty degrees
- Feet are fully supported by the floor
- Back is fully supported with appropriate lumbar support when sitting vertical or leaning back slightly
- Thighs and hips are supported by a well-padded seat and generally parallel to the floor

- Knees are about the same height as the hips with the feet slightly forward

As with general ergonomic principles, these computer workstation guidelines are more difficult for us to abide by. Specifically, low chairs cause our knees to be above our pelvis, forcing the hips into greater flexion, and low desks and monitors encourage us to lean forward. Both of these may lead to a deviation from neutral spine posture. There are some desks and chairs that are more tall-friendly than others, and these should be sought out. However, some simple adaptations can help. First, the chair can be raised either with extra-large casters or a longer pneumatic cylinder. Second, furniture raisers can increase the work surface height (these are also useful for raising couches and other furniture). Third, monitor stands can bring the monitor to a height that encourages neutral neck posture. Lastly, extra-large computer mice better suit our larger hands.

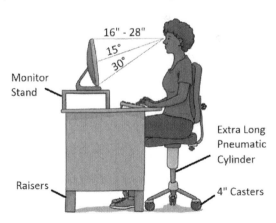

One particularly challenging ergonomic situation is the classroom. I remember well how incredibly uncomfortable those desks were. Evidently tall kids in general tend to experience this as they're found to have more desk related back pain.[29]

A few adaptations could help a lot. Perhaps the simplest would be a slanted, raised work surface. But I can understand how this might be a bit difficult what with the pressure to conform. It wasn't until grad school that I tossed caution to the wind and started bringing my raised work surface and kneeling chair to my exams.

Another issue I'd like to mention is that people often incorrectly equate comfort with cushions and bells and whistles; the more padding and features a chair has, the better people think it is. Perhaps these things help, but it's far more important that a chair fits the individual.

A more general recommendation for people of all heights that's ever more frequently being made is to do less sitting. It's for this reason that sit-stand desks, treadmill desks, and routines that regularly interject movement are becoming increasingly popular. That being said, there are times when reclining in something like a zero gravity chair for certain tasks such as reading can be a time to rest an aching back.

I was in graduate school with a ton of work to do and a dissertation hanging over my head right when my back was at its worst. So I was desperate to find a position I could get work done from that didn't make my back worse. What I learned though was that there's no one ideal position. So I built a setup that let me work from a variety of positions including zero gravity, sitting, and standing. The key to working in the zero gravity position is a touchpad keyboard. An obvious problem with the setup is that it probably wouldn't fly in most workplaces. A more professional solution that allows for a similar set of positions is the Altwork. But it's expensive and I'm not sure if it would be suitable for tall people.

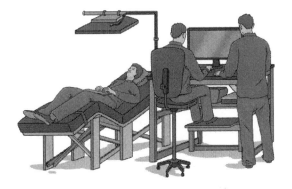

Cars

In the previous chapter, I provided some tips on selecting a tall-friendly car, specifically by looking for a large Vision Line Height. Beyond this though, there are some modifications that can be made. Note, however, that any kind of modification may have insurance, safety, and/or legal implications, so modify at your own risk. That being said, not modifying can also be hazardous.

First, there are seat modifications. Custom or aftermarket seat brackets, like those by ExtendMySeat, can be installed to gain extra legroom and sometimes headroom. An alternative method for lowering the seat is to remove padding from the seat cushion. For the seat back, as with other seats like those on airplanes, I have found a small cushion works well as a higher and larger lumbar support. Then there are aftermarket seats. The best one for us is probably the Vario XXL by Greiner, which was actually designed with tall people in mind.

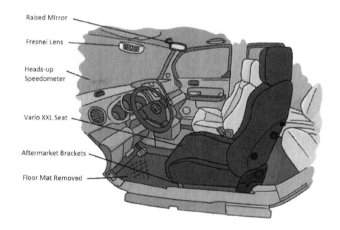

Raised Mirror

Fresnel Lens

Heads-up Speedometer

Vario XXL Seat

Aftermarket Brackets

Floor Mat Removed

Next are modifications to compensate for the legroom/reach discrepancy that I explained in the previous chapter. Telescopic steering wheels and pedals help with this. Beyond these, a mobility shop can extend steering wheels either with secondary wheels or column extensions, the latter of which are rare and pricey.

As far as visibility goes, lowering the seat is the most effective thing you can do. However, this can be uncomfortable as it effectively decreases legroom. There are a few other alternative modifications that can help. First, rear view mirrors can be repositioned higher on the windshield or even mounted on the roof so they don't block line of sight. Second, the problem of the steering wheel blocking view of the speedometer can be solved via an auxiliary heads-up speedometer or GPS that gives speed. Third, a Fresnel lens on the windshield may be useful for seeing traffic lights normally blocked by the roof. Perhaps another way to see some traffic lights is through the sunroof. Rather humorously, I once tried to install a sunroof for this very purpose only to find my head just stuck out entirely. I don't recommend this.

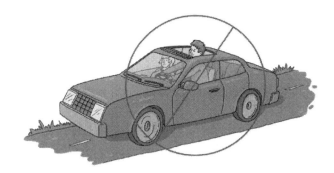

One final tip is to remove the floor mats. I find it surprising how much extra legroom this creates. Driving barefoot does similarly, though may not be legal, nor comfortable for some.

Some of the above modifications might require the assistance of a mobility shop. However, the more careful shops may not be willing to help, as insurance companies may require any modifications to be approved through a lengthy process that may require crash testing.

Bikes

In addition to being a sport, cycling is becoming an ever more popular alternative mode of transportation as it's cheap, provides exercise, and doesn't pollute. Tall people have yet another motivation, namely the ergonomic superiority of bikes over cars and public transit.

This superiority arises from the fact that bikes are both available in multiple sizes and are adjustable, plus they have unlimited headroom. Yet there are still some points that I'd like to mention in the context of this chapter.

Many brands have sizes all way up to 64cm. My 64cm Surly Cross-Check works pretty well for me. If you look around, you can find 66cm and even 68cm bikes. What a lot of these have in common though is that they still use standard sized pedal cranks. And while this will be OK for casual riders, others will prefer more proportional cranks. One study found optimum crank length to be approximately twenty percent of leg length.[60]

A good analogy is jumping. You wouldn't tell a taller basketball player not to bend his knees as much, right? Likewise, cranks should allow a cyclist's hips and knees to move through a similar range of motion independent of stature. This seems fairly intuitive. Yet a lot of average height cyclists still balk at the idea of taller riders needing longer cranks. I suggest installing some children's tricycle cranks on their bikes to prove a point.

The problem with longer cranks though is that they may require slightly different frame geometry, including a higher bottom bracket to avoid clipping a pedal on the ground. This can be achieved with a custom frame, such as those designed by Lennard Zinn. These can be a bit pricey. Luckily, Zinn has also designed a few more affordable stock bikes for taller riders, the Big Apple, Flite 747, and KHS BNT 29er. I rode the 747 for a while myself and can tell you it's a fantastic bike. Another company called DirtySixer is pushing the envelope for wheel size. While 29" has typically been the largest wheel diameter on bikes specifically for tall people, DirtySixer is stepping this up to 36".

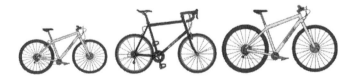

The tall cyclist is also likely heavier than average and thus should pay special attention to frame strength and stiffness and the quality of the various components, such as the braking mechanisms. As far as frame material goes, steel and titanium have an advantage over aluminum in that they won't fatigue as long as stresses remain below a certain limit. I don't mean to say that an aluminum frame properly designed for the rider can't make an excellent solution. We do make airplanes out of aluminum after all. As some might argue though, airplanes are retired after a certain number of years, which may not be the case for bikes.

Doors and Doorways

I like the expression "dumb as a doorknob" because I think doorknobs really are some of the dumbest things around. They're ideal for one height and one height only. For everyone else, and this will be most true for tall people, unnecessary torque is applied to the spine.

Regulations specify doorknob heights between 2'10" and 4'.[61] While the upper end of this range would be suitable for moderately tall people, the mid-range is far more common. Besides the additional torque, this can encourage us to deviate from a neutral spine posture. We can compensate by reducing our height with a slight lunge.

Even dumber than doorknobs are doorways. Unlike doorknobs, higher doorways have no adverse effect on the average person. So there's no excuse for making them so low! Furthermore, we often make them lower than the 6'8" height specified in regulations.[61]

While ducking under a doorway may appear inconsequential at a first glance, doing so dozens of times a day and by slouching is yet another harmful practice for the spine. Once again though, we can adapt by flexing the ankles, hips, and knees rather than the spine, creating a slight drop as we cross the threshold. It's also helpful to cross the threshold halfway between steps, where stature is effectively the lowest.

Lastly, the extremely tall among us should watch out for those massive protruding sharp metal hinges on commercial doorways—those things are potentially lethal.

Bedroom

When I hit my growth spurt, my mom most kindly got me an extra-long twin bed (39" x 80"). Nowadays, I sleep on a queen (60" x 80"). This length gives me one inch to spare, for which I'm most grateful. Perhaps when I buy a new bed someday, though, I'll get a California king (72" x 84"). Those who need longer will have to go with custom.

One great place to get extra-long beds and bedding, and other tall things for that matter, is Tall Paul's Tall Mall. A really neat product they sell is called an Extend-a-Bed. Basically, a board hangs out from between the box spring and mattress. It's supported by legs and a foam block sits on top of it, thereby extending the bed. Another helpful tall solution is the bed raiser, making it easier to get in and out of bed, plus creating a larger space to store things.

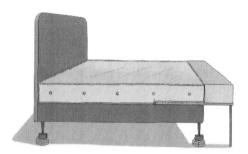

Bathroom

The bathroom is yet another shared space that presents many ergonomic challenges. Low shower heads in particular are one of our greatest gripes. Yet they also happen to be one of the easiest to adapt. Adjustable height sliding shower heads, overhead rain shower heads, and pivoting and s-style shower head extension arms can all effectively solve this problem.

Another helpful addition is a curved shower rod, which keeps the shower curtain at a greater distance from our elbows when washing our hair. And for bathing, drain covers allow the water to fill to a greater depth.

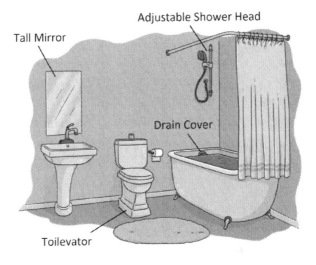

Adjustable Shower Head

Tall Mirror

Drain Cover

Toilevator

Mirrors can be raised or simply tilted to accommodate us. Finally, toilets can be raised via a Toilevator, raised seat, or with a wall mounted toilet at any desired height. However, I'd like to note that we evolved defecating from a squat position which tends to better open up the anorectal angle,[62] thereby easing abdominal pressure and decreasing risk of hemorrhoids, this on top of decreasing defecation time.[63] In light of this, relatively low toilets might not be such a bad thing after all.

For bathrooms that cannot be adapted, our interactions can instead be adapted. For example, a squat can be used to permit a neutral spine posture while flushing the toilette, washing your hands, or looking in the mirror.

Curiously, toilet raisers are actually intended for elderly people, not tall people. This is because they enable standing up from a seated position with lesser exertion and are easier on the low back. But now consider the scenario where you have a tall **and** elderly person. They would benefit from an even greater rise.

The elderly benefit from many adaptive aids, and most of these, like the toilet raiser, should be scaled up for tall elderly people. These include canes, walkers, and wheelchairs. And beyond this, given the greater frailty that comes with age, all of the other adaptations I've described so far become all that much more important.

Elderly people are more likely to end up in hospitals and other medical centers. These are designed for near average height people, from the sinks, to the beds, and even the operating rooms. The tall elderly person may require multiple aids to be moved. Medical devices such as braces, prosthetics, catheters, and surgical implants may not be large enough nor strong enough.

It's best for an aging tall person to remain in an environment in which they have the freedom to adapt. Easier said than done, but as the old adage goes, aging is not for the faint of heart.

Jobs

For tall people on the job, the combination of poor ergonomics, pressure to perform, and repetitive tasks makes for a high risk of injury. Tasks like being a cashier may seem harmless at a first glance. However, holding poor posture to work at a low surface for long hours day after day is sure to lead to injury. Note that those rubber standing mats may worsen matters by effectively increasing our height. Now consider the tasks that are renowned for being hard on the body, like operating a jack hammer. By adding heavy lifting and vibration into the mix, injury is a near certainty.

The best jobs for us, in an ergonomics sense, are the flexible ones. For example, if the tall cashier is allowed to intermittently sit on a swiveling stool, then some of the risk may be mitigated. In general, if we're allowed to adapt the job to our needs, then there usually is a way to make the job safer.

There are of course jobs where little can be done. A submarine officer, for one, is stuck with low ceilings. It's often jobs like these that have height limits though. The US army has a height limit of 6'8" while NASA's restrictions are more stringent at 6'3" for commanders and pilots.[64,65] I sincerely apologize if I just discouraged anyone.

Desk work has become the most common ergonomic scenario. And though desk work is far from ideal from a health standpoint, we shouldn't be much worse off than average height people if we adopt effective adaptations.

Clothing and Footwear

Clothing can play a role in ergonomics. For example, protective clothing allows the wearer to hold a load close to the body, thereby reducing the torque acting about the spine. Such functions of clothing are present in many physical jobs like firefighting and construction working. When our clothing fits poorly, risk of injury increases.

But in the context of tall stature, our more common complaint with clothing relates to aesthetics. So, we would benefit from learning to do a couple basic alterations. The first is taking in the sides on an overly baggy shirt. The second is stretching shirts to increase their length. It's also helpful to air-dry rather than use the dryer. I learned this the hard way, to my extreme frustration. Somewhat less critical yet still helpful is to wash in cold water.[50] Wearing, on the other hand, increases the width of shirts. Though avoiding this of course would defeat their purpose.

As far as footwear goes, besides size, another important consideration is how much it increases our stature. High heels and dress shoes, for instance, increase stature for social purposes, which can be important. But in a biomechanical context, this makes little sense. Furthermore, for tall people, it's surely detrimental as ergonomic issues increase in parallel with height. For example, an inch of heel height reduces legroom in the car and puts that kitchen counter even further from elbow height. So, outside of certain social contexts, we would be better off with shoes that do not significantly increase stature. Useful terms when searching for such shoes include 'flats' and 'zero drop'.

Social Situations

The interactions considered in the field of ergonomics don't usually include those with another person. Yet when two people of significantly different heights interact, the principles of ergonomics become relevant.

It's taken me many years and a lot of back pain to recognize that I adopt terrible posture when interacting with much shorter people. This is particularly true when it's a superior or a person of 'great stature'. How I do this is by slouching in the spine and sagging into one hip. I imagine it looks as bad as it feels. But when I stand erect, it can sometimes be a bit awkward and in noisy environments I have trouble hearing.

I've since learned a few tricks. I often find a lower ground, such as presented by a staircase, to stand. Other times I find a place to sit. It can be somewhat humorous when you're the same height as a shorter person despite the fact that you're sitting. Another option is to lean backwards or sideways into a wall—whatever it takes to keep that spine straight. All this probably seems fairly obvious, yet if you spectate at a social gathering, you'll likely notice the tallest people doing a lot of slouching.

Mindset

Now that I've explained some tall solutions, there are a few issues relating to mindset that I'd like to address. Firstly, I've been told by many people that it's too much of an endeavor to build some adaptations. What such people need to understand though is that, while it does take work, it's a onetime thing that will benefit you for years to come. And when you do succeed, this thwarting of society's will to shrink you brings a sense of renegade accomplishment, a sense of sticking it to the man.

People also commonly feel that adapting requires additional ongoing work, such as for putting a stool in place each time you do the dishes or wash the vegetables. However, people in the developed world tend to error on the side of too little energy expenditure, increasing the risk of disease. So please think of this additional effort as a way of interjecting movement into daily life. The greater challenge is mustering the willpower. Once it becomes habit though, it's no different from brushing your teeth.

The next issue pertains to the alternatives to adapting that I've heard people commonly suggest. One alternative is to simply ask others to do the troublesome tasks. However, were we to heed such advice, we would really limit ourselves, as so many interactions with manufactured objects are compromised by tall stature. Besides, it's a matter of pride to carry out one's own chores such as shoveling the driveway, doing the dishes, cutting the grass, and driving the car.

The second alternative I often hear proposed is to just deal with it. In other words, accept that these deficient interactions are going to cause injury, and await the inevitable. For every instance of this suggestion, I come across multiple instances of tall people complaining of back pain and other injuries.

There's a serious need to raise awareness for our increased risk of injuries and also for some solutions. I address this and other social issues in the final chapter of this book. Before then though, in the next chapter, I explore how tall people become tall in the first place.

GROWTH

"The Gentle Giant"

—8'11" Robert Pershing Wadlow

This book is all about being tall. But how does one become tall? And how can we predict this? These are the main questions I answer in this chapter. I also summarize some height related disorders, briefly recognize some of the world's tallest people, and explore the bizarre business of intentionally shrinking people. First though, is a summary of the physiological processes that lead to growth.

Growing Up

Tall stature, more than any other physical characteristic, gets a lot of comments. Most of the time people want to know how tall you are. Occasionally, though, someone asks the peculiar question of how you **became** so tall. It's almost as if they think you sat down and wrote a prolific business plan. Obviously, you didn't.

But growth is nevertheless kind of like a business—a business run by hormones. And like with any other business, there's a pecking order. There are the executives that rule, the managers that carry out their bidding, and then the workers who do the heavy lifting:

- Executive: Growth-hormone-releasing hormone (GHRH)
- Executive: Growth-hormone-inhibiting hormone (GHIH)
- Managers: Human growth hormone (HGH)
- Workers: Insulin like growth factor (IGF-1)

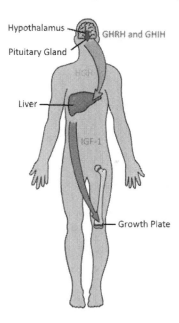

The heavy lifting of the workers (IGF-1) is to travel throughout the body triggering growth. This includes the growth plates of the bones, thereby increasing the dimensions of the body.

This hormone business is booming at birth but then declines from there, except for a brief surge in the teenage years known as a growth spurt. It's at this point where the height related comments really ramp up. After the growth spurt, the growth plates close (fuse) as indirectly caused by all the sex hormones. This usually occurs by age fifteen for girls and seventeen for boys.

By that point, we'll be taller than just about everyone around us. And we may begin to reflect and wonder how we got into this agreeable yet sometimes challenging circumstance.

Both genetics and environment are behind this, nature and nurture if you will. The genetic contribution is commonly thought to be responsible for between sixty and eighty percent of height variation among individuals.[66]

To visualize genes, I think the human genome book analogy is helpful, as in the illustration below. Each cell in the human body contains at least one copy of this genome book in a space about the size of the head of a pin.

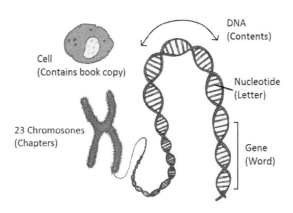

Cell
(Contains book copy)

DNA
(Contents)

Nucleotide
(Letter)

23 Chromosones
(Chapters)

Gene
(Word)

Imagine that a mom and dad each write a book for their child. Each of these books has thirty-three chapters that tell the child what to do with their life, kind of like a manual. For most of these parallel books, duplicate content is covered, just with different parenting styles. But in the final pair of chapters, which together dictate gender, mum and dad take different approaches entirely. Mothers are OK with a boy or a girl. Fathers, on the other hand, are decisive.

In more technical terms, the final chromosome from the female is always an X while for the male it's either an X or a Y. If the result is two X chromosomes then the gender is female, whereas an X coupled with a Y yields a male.

Because of the duplication of chromosomes, the genes are also duplicated. A gene that prevails as the active gene is considered dominant while the other is considered recessive. Though a gene may be inactive, it can still be passed on to offspring. For example, my balding is far more advanced than my father's was at my age, and this is likely because I've inherited the associated genes from my mother's side, despite the fact that she herself has a full head of hair.

The genes affecting human height are multiple (polygenic). As genetic investigations become ever more advanced, researchers are finding new genes that influence height with the count now at over four hundred.[67] These genes affect height by, among other ways, influencing the secretion of HGH and IGF-1.

As far as environmental factors go, these include childhood stress, illness, temperature, activities, and nutrition. Nutrition has the biggest influence at a young age. High protein intake, such as from milk, in particular is linked with tall stature.[68,69] I, for one, drank a lot of milk when I was growing up.

Nutrition and other environmental factors affect not just the individual, but future generations as they impact epigenetics (the expression of genes). If you think of genetics as hardware, then epigenetics is like software. So just like you can update the apps on your device, your epigenetics can become altered over the course of your lifetime. And though epigenetics are only thought to pervade over a finite number of generations, evidence is gathering that these changes are the catalyst to the more traditional evolutionary adaptations driven by natural selection.

It's interesting to consider the Dutch, of whom I share a quarter of my ancestry, in this context. Dutch height has increased by about eight inches over the last one hundred fifty years as they soared past Americans.[70] And this has nothing to do with their trying to keep their heads above water. Rather, it's thought this is due to environmental factors. More recently, however, Dutch height has been tapering off. This is likely because their genes have nearly maximized their height potential. If a famine were to arrive now, it would take several generations to reverse this epigenetic change. However, if prosperous times continue, the genes will adjust to reflect the current height, leaving room for even greater stature via epigenetic changes.

Now that we've established how we grow to be so tall, the next logical question relates to why we're so rare. I'm sure you've noticed our scarcity in large public gatherings, but have you ever really thought about why there are more average height people than tall people?

To explain our rarity, let's get back to nutrition for a moment. Picture it as a six-sided die, where a six represents abundant nutrition and a one abysmal. You have an equal probability of rolling any number from one through six. So if growth was affected by only nutrition, then there would be just as many people my height as there are average height people.

But there are many other factors, such as our various genes. So let's picture another six-sided die as a single gene, with a six representing the full expression of the gene. Now roll it with the nutrition die. Notice how there's only one way to roll a height maximizing sum of twelve. Similarly, there's only one way to roll a height minimizing sum of two. In contrast, there are six different ways to roll a sum of seven. So by having two dice, we're more likely to end up with an average sum. Adding more dice into the mix further establishes this relationship. Similarly, the great number of independent variables affecting height means that there are more average height people than tall or short people.

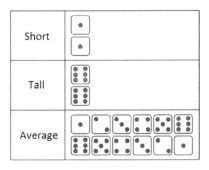

By now you should be pretty familiar with the business of growth, and also why we're so uncommon. So the next time someone asks how you became so tall, perhaps you can share with them your rather irreproducible business plan.

Predicting and Quantifying Human Height

By receiving a combination of genes from both parents, a child will tend to grow up to be about their parents' gender adjusted average height. This leads to the simplest method of estimating adult height: Take the average height of the parents and add two and a half inches for boys or subtract the same for girls.[71] But if the child's height trajectory points to an unexpected height, don't go hunting down the mailman just yet; with so many genes involved, some of which may have been recessive, and the possibility of environmental influences, a child's eventual adult height can differ considerably from parental height. I'm a perfect example of this given I'm about a half a foot taller than would have been expected from my parents' heights.

Another simple approach to predicting adult height may be more accurate in this regard, which is to double a boy's height at age two or a girl's height at age one and a half.[71] A more advanced approach is the Khamis-Roche method, which I use in the height calculator on www.Tall.Life. The most advanced methods use bone age which can be estimated from X-rays.

The last approach I'll mention is to determine a child's height percentile and then check the corresponding adult height for that same percentile. Percentiles can be determined from growth charts or height percentile calculators. Note that a height percentile is simply the percentage of people in a group that are shorter. The remainder, of course, are taller.

So percentiles can also be useful for quantifying just how tall you are. In the extremes of height, though, percentiles become less useful as they're all between ninety-nine and one hundred percent. Instead, it's more telling to consider the number of standard deviations above average. A standard deviation from average, as shown below, is about three inches.

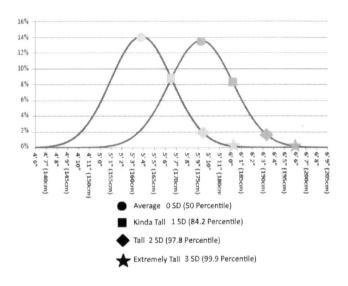

● Average 0 SD (50 Percentile)

■ Kinda Tall 1 SD (84.2 Percentile)

◆ Tall 2 SD (97.8 Percentile)

★ Extremely Tall 3 SD (99.9 Percentile)

No matter what approach to predicting adult height you use, it helps to keep a record through the years. My mother used a doorframe for this purpose, which worked out great until she ran out of door frame.

In rare cases, a prediction for stature significantly above parental height can be a sign that there's an underlying disorder.

Disorders and Syndromes Related to Tall Stature

The following summary of somewhat rare height related disorders is merely for raising awareness. For anything more than that, specialists such as geneticists, endocrinologists, and pediatricians should be consulted. If you want to do some research on your own, you might start with the following two open access articles:

- *Investigation and management of tall stature*
- *Tall stature in children: differential diagnosis and management*

Chromosome Disorders

As I explained earlier, humans typically have twenty-three pairs of chromosomes with the final pair consisting of either an XX (female) or XY (male) combination. Occasionally, however, the male sperm and/or female egg may have additional X or Y chromosomes that get passed on to the child. The most well-known result is Klinefelter (XXY). The extra chromosome may trigger additional growth.[72]

Other Genetic Disorders

Besides an abnormal number of chromosomes, there are other genetic disorders that can cause tall stature.

Marfan's Syndrome is the one we hear the most about. It affects human connective tissue and commonly presents with a long and slender build and excess joint mobility. Below are some other height related genetic disorders (overgrowth syndromes):

- Sotos' Syndrome
- Weaver's Syndrome
- Marshall–Smith Syndrome
- Beckwith–Wiedemann Syndrome
- Multiple Endocrine Neoplasia
- ACTH Resistance
- Homocysteinuria

Endocrine Disorders

The endocrine consists of the glands that deliver hormones to other organs in the body via direct secretion into the circulatory system. Disorders of the endocrine can affect growth as follows:

- **Growth Hormone Disorders** - In some people, excess HGH is secreted by the pituitary gland. Most often this is due to a benign tumor. This excess hormone increases rate of growth. When it occurs during childhood, it may result in gigantism. When it occurs after puberty, the condition is known as acromegaly. Often, large hands, face, and feet are present with gigantism. Both the tallest recorded man, 8'11"

Robert Wadlow, and woman, 8'2" Zeng Jinlian, had gigantism.

- **Delayed or Advanced Puberty** - Testosterone and estrogen affect growth hormone production as well as the onset and duration of puberty. High levels of these sex hormones may cause an early (precocious) puberty, thereby early tall stature followed by stunted growth. Low levels of sex hormone may delay puberty, allowing the growth plates to remain open and resulting in tall adult stature.
- **Hyperthyroidism** - The thyroid is a gland in the neck that's responsible for regulating the rate of living, essentially. An overactive thyroid can lead to increased growth.

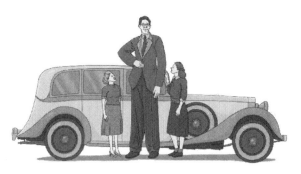

The World's Tallest People

What is truly remarkable about height is just how relative it is. For instance, at about one foot above average height, I generally feel like I'm the tallest person around. But the fact is there are a lot of people who are a foot taller than me. And then there are people who are yet another foot taller! Unless you're 8'3" Sultan Kösen or 7'3" Sun Fang, there's always a taller man or woman, respectively.

Also relative are the challenges we face. For instance, I have often complained about clothes not fitting and cars being too small. But compared to the truly tallest people, I really don't have much to complain about. The tallest people also struggle the most with social and health issues. The latter is partly due to the fact that this extraordinary stature often comes from disorders such as gigantism.

Even more extraordinary than their height are the stories of adventure and perseverance behind these friendly giants. Really, these champions of height deserve far more recognition than this short section provides. Perhaps if there's a second edition of this book then I'll devote a chapter to the world's tallest people. For now, I'd like to give a quick shout-out to two of the world's tallest people who most graciously agreed to take a read of this book, 7'8" Abdramane Dembele and 7'8" George Bell.

Stunting Growth

While tall stature confers many advantages, there comes a height at which the cons outweigh the pros. When such extreme stature is due to an underlying disorder, then it's this that's usually treated. However, if it's merely familial, there are procedures for reducing eventual adult stature.

The earliest methods involved the surgical shortening of the femurs or the more strategic destroying of the growth plates.[73] Besides being exceedingly painful and risky, an obvious issue with such procedures is that proportions are distorted. Additionally, leg length discrepancies may result.

It's no surprise then that, upon their introduction, drug interventions were readily embraced. Sex steroids including etinyloestradiol, a type of estrogen, and testosterone act to prematurely end puberty, thereby leading to the early fusing of growth plates and the halting of growth. When administered before puberty (usually around ten years for girls and twelve and a half years for boys), expected reduction in final height is a little under three inches.[74]

Though such drug interventions remain the predominant approach to this day, they have their drawbacks. In particular, there may be an increased risk of cancer[75] and estrogen treatment has been reported to cause some fertility issues.[76] This is ironic given the common justification for restricting a girl's height has been to improve her chances of finding a partner to have children with.

A drug that does not affect puberty that has been used is a synthetic version of somatostatin (GHIH). However, a 2006 study found this not to be as effective as sex steroid treatment.[77]

As I mentioned earlier, genetics is thought to account for sixty to eighty percent of height variability. The remainder is due to environmental factors such as nutrition. Curiously, I found nothing about limiting nutrition in the literature on stunting growth. I think it's fairly obvious though that avoiding excess nutrition is an important first step.

A potential future approach for capping adult height is gene therapy. Gene therapy was first used on humans in the 1990s[78] and is rapidly becoming more popular. Therapeutic DNA is delivered into the cells, replacing faulty genes, essentially. Gene therapy has largely been used for treating diseases, though enhancement is another use.[79] Gene therapy may eventually be used for treating height related disorders as well as extreme familial tall stature.[79] However, the vast array of genes that affect height does present enormous challenges.

Women have been the primary recipient of height reduction treatments, with social issues being the predominant justification. The 1950s saw the most unrestrained treatment, beginning with girls with predicted heights as close to average as 5'8".[80] This peak in treatment was due to the strict gender rules of the 1950s, where great emphasis was placed on a women's finding a husband and raising children. In the decades that followed, however, gender rules loosened and women increasingly found their way into the workplace, where height confers its many advantages. Today, the use of height reduction treatments is far more conservative, reserved mostly for women above 6'. Given there's still some dismantling of gender rules to be done, it's likely this threshold will increase.

Furthermore, while tall stature has been shown to lead to such adverse psychological outcomes as depression, one study found that height reduction treatment does not improve matters.[81] Some opponents to height reduction therapy even suggest that this 'medicalization' of tall stature, where it's something that must be treated, does more harm than good.[80]

I discuss such social issues as these further in the final chapter. Beyond social issues, however, there's an arguably more significant drawback of extreme tall stature, and that has to do with longevity, which is the topic of the next chapter.

CHAPTER 7

LONGEVITY

"... it is a general rule that the larger live longer than the smaller ..."

—Aristotle

Tall stature is generally associated with good health. Both require a descent standard of living, particularly good nutrition, after all. Also, there's a general trend in nature where larger animals live longer. Recently though, there's mounting evidence that tall people are at increased risk for some diseases, namely cancers and atrial fibrillation. Further, some researchers are concluding that shorter people live longer. In actuality, there's likely an optimum height for the greatest longevity.

I've devoted the first section of this chapter to explaining all this. While I think this will fascinate most readers while raising awareness, some might wish to cut to the chase and read the Perspective and Prevention section first.

Tall Stature, Disease, and Longevity

Seeing as tall people are rather rare, the medical world doesn't devote much attention to the effect our height has on our health. We're considered negligible outliers for the most part. The exception to this is the basketball stars among us—when world famous former basketball players start dropping like flies, people start to ask questions.

An obvious hypothesis is that their grueling athletic careers are to blame. But when you look at athletes in most other sports, you don't see this trend. Instead, it's becoming apparent that basketball players' extraordinary height—commonly over 7' in the NBA— might have something to do with it.

In hopes of getting to the bottom of this, the *National Basketball Players Association* began a screening program in 2015.[82] What was found was an unusually high prevalence for signs of heart disease. And with many former players suffering from heart arrhythmias, such as the most vocal 6'9" Larry Bird, and heart related deaths, a picture does start to take shape. Former players also seem to have a bad habit of developing cancer, including 7'2" Kareem Abdul-Jabbar. And the plethora of musculoskeletal injuries doesn't make life easier either, as 6'11" Bill Walton has written about at length in his book, *Back from the Dead*.

All this will probably be puzzling to most people, as we usually associate height with good health. Perhaps this is because the only way to grow tall is with a nurturing environment. And some studies actually do find that taller people are better off, particularly for heart problems.[83–85] This may be due to the fact that we tend to have leaner bodies and that our larger caliber blood vessels (arteries, veins, and capillaries) are not as sensitive to atherosclerosis (buildup of plaque).[83] Perhaps it's only in the extreme heights typical of NBA big men that the cons outweigh the pros for heart disease.

Another reason why we might expect tall people to live longer is that there's a general trend in nature of increasing lifespan with size. This trend was recognized as far back as 350 BC by Aristotle.[86] But what is the explanation for it?

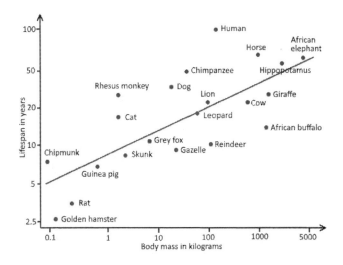

Consider that animals of all sizes, from a mouse up to an elephant, tend to have a similar number of heart beats in a lifetime. This is somewhere on the order of a billion.[87] But because the relatively stronger hearts (square-cube law) of small animals beat faster, they use up these billion beats in a shorter period of time and so don't live as long. This concept of using up heart beats is an oversimplification and I hope it doesn't mislead you into becoming a couch potato—that would be most unhealthy. Nevertheless, the implication that life is something that's used up does have some validity.

Beyond heart rate, a better measure of the rate at which animals live is metabolic rate (rate of energy expenditure). Larger animals require more energy and so have higher metabolic rates. Yet in relation to mass, they actually have lower metabolic rates as per the square-cube law. In turn, this relatively lower metabolic rate coincides with greater longevity. Max Rubner dubbed this The Rate of Living Theory, where larger animals live more gradually and thereby longer.[88]

Where this trend starts to fall apart, though, is within species. The classic example is dogs. Small breed dogs live fifteen to sixteen years while the largest breeds, Mastiffs for example, live only seven to eight years. In addition to heart disease, another potential end game is cancer. And given tall people also tend to be at higher risk of cancer, this warrants the following brief summary of it.

Our bodies are made up of trillions of cells. All of these cells eventually die and so have to be replaced by new ones. Ordinarily, there's a balance between the formation of new cells and the dying off of old cells. However, mutations to a cell's DNA can alter this regulation such that uncontrolled cell growth and division can occur, causing cancer essentially. A couple sources for mutations include random errors during cell splitting and carcinogens.

It only takes one cell mutation for a cancer to begin. And given tall people have more cells, it's no surprise then that we're at increased risk of cancer. For further appreciation of this, consider that we consume more food and water, breath more air, and have more skin facing the sun, and thereby expose ourselves to more potential carcinogens.[89],[90]

If increased size is such a problem for cancer, then one would expect that larger species would be at increased risk of cancer. But they aren't. The largest animals on Earth, whales, for example, actually have lower cancer rates than humans.[91] This is known as Peto's Paradox.[92]

The explanation for Peto's Paradox draws on evolutionary theory; natural selection has led larger species to adapt for their greater number of cells by developing coping mechanisms against cancer. This includes larger cells that don't split as often,[93] more gradual growth and thereby aging pathways, fewer endogenous retroviruses,[94] and unique genetic adaptations.[95]

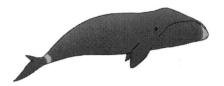

Tall people have not benefitted from this same extent of evolutionary adaptation and the result is a higher risk of cancer. Many studies confirm this. In a *National Institutes of Health* study with a cohort of over half a million, it was found that increased height correlated with increased risk of cancer nearly across the board.[68] In general, a four inch increase in height yielded a five percent increased risk of cancer for men and eight percent for women. This is somewhat low in comparison to another study with a similar sized cohort; a two inch increase in height corresponded with an increased risk of four percent and seven percent for men and women for cancer and three percent for both for death from cancer.[90]

Studies also confirm that we're at higher risk for an arrhythmia known as atrial fibrillation, a rapid and irregular heart beat originating from electrical disturbances in the upper chambers of the heart. One study found a four inch increase in height coincided with a thirty percent increased risk of atrial fibrillation[96] and another found that for every six inches above average, there's a fifty percent increase in risk.[97] Atrial fibrillation is estimated to be the cause of more than fifteen percent of all strokes.[98]

Ironically, procedures for correcting atrial fibrillation are designed for average height people and may not be as successful or even possible for extremely tall people. Deeper chest cavities can decrease the effect of cardioversions, catheters may be too short for ablations, and surgical tools may not be long enough for keyhole surgery.

So, does all this mean that to be tall is to live short? Thomas Samaras of *Reventropy Associates* thinks so. He has pulled together the extensive literature contributing to this topic and found that, while there are many studies demonstrating increasing longevity with height, these tend to insufficiently account for the effects of increasing socioeconomic status with height among other confounding factors.[99] He estimates that 1.3 years are lost for every inch increase in height.

But regardless of whether shorter people live longer or not, if they do it's common sense that there'd be a limit to this trend. In actuality, the height-longevity relationship should be nonlinear and upside-down U-shaped such that there exists an optimum height. Evolutionary theory would suggest that this optimum height be somewhere near average height; longevity is an important factor for the propagation of the human species, and if those with the greatest longevity differed in height greatly from average, the average height would trend towards this height.

Perspective and Prevention

It's possible that the tallest of people, with all else being equal, tend to not live as long as average height people. But not everything is equal. For example, taller people tend to have higher socioeconomic status and this correlates with greater longevity. Many other factors come into play and the overall physiological impact of height on longevity is small. Thomas Samaras himself recognizes this as he states his caveat which is that height is responsible for merely ten percent of the overall longevity picture.[100]

In fact, genetics in general are thought to play a small role in the overall longevity picture, approximately twenty-five percent as demonstrated in twin studies.[101] Instead, it's increasingly being recognized that it's lifestyle factors that are more critical.[102] This is true for nutrition in particular for its role in cancer. Poor nutrition can actually cause cancer, while good nutrition can prevent and aid in the recovery from cancer. And given increased nutrition has been one explanation for increasing risk of cancer with stature,[89] this warrants the following points.

The foods most widely cited for their role in preventing cancer are fruits and vegetables. In addition to vitamins, minerals, and fiber, these contain phytochemicals, of which there are thousands of varieties. Phytochemicals afford plants their ability to fight off threats including germs, fungi, and bugs. When consumed by humans, these same phytochemicals play a role in preventing cancer. This is by preventing damage to DNA and by slowing the growth of and killing off of cancer cells. These benefits are perhaps one reason why such prominent entities as the *American Cancer Society* and *World Health Organization* are increasingly recommending more plant food in our diets. Some foods widely recognized for these benefits, including in an accessible book entitled *Foods That Fight Cancer*,[103] are as follows:

- Cruciferous vegetables including brussels sprouts, broccoli, and kale
- Herbs and spices including turmeric
- Members of the allium family including garlic and onions
- Fruits including berries and citrus
- Tomatoes particularly when concentrated such as in paste or sauce
- Many nuts and seeds
- Legumes including soy
- Japanese green tea
- Red wine in moderation
- Dark chocolate.
- Foods high in Omega-3 like some fish, walnuts, flax, and chia seeds

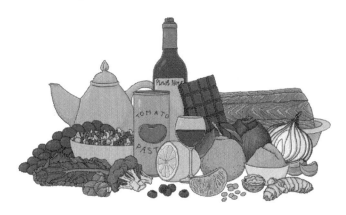

Other important dietary considerations include avoiding trans fats and processed foods, minimizing saturated fats, salt, and sugar, and staying hydrated. A memorable quote on this topic that's found in a highly praised book on nutrition, entitled *In Defense of Foods*, is, "Eat food. Not too much. Mostly plants".[104]

Beyond food, it's also critical to get enough exercise, movement throughout the day, and sufficient rest. And we should avoid smoking, excess drinking, and drugs. Finally, how we function in society is also important for our health. It's the combination of all of these lifestyle factors that affects our longevity, as demonstrated by the long lived Okinawans of Japan.

It's also important to not overdue things. Anecdotally, when my great grandfather was asked how he lived to ninety-seven years of age, he replied, "Moderation in all things". Aristotle called this the golden mean, while in Buddhism it's referred to as the middle path.

There's a variety of medical professionals that can assist on this topic. Nutritionists, dieticians, and naturopaths can help in coming up with a diet tailored to the individual. Various exercise professionals can help with an exercise plan. And a variety of doctors, starting with a general practitioner, can spot diseases in their early stages, providing for an opportunity to intervene with changes to lifestyle as well as with modern medicine.

The Future of Longevity

Western science is increasingly recognizing the role of lifestyle in longevity, and guidelines are reflecting this.

Additionally, medical advancements are being made at a breathtaking rate and these may thwart the diseases that shorten lifespans, including those that are more prevalent in tall people. Soon, genetic therapies, including for cancers, will become commonplace. Perhaps these will be learned from studying larger long-lived species like elephants and whales. Custom artificial organ replacement will also become common, even for the heart. These advancements will be the equalizers among people of all heights.

In the not so distant future, our lifespans will be less determined by the genetics we're born with—though these too will be controlled—and more by other factors such as financial assets and simply our decision for how long to live. Some people are predicting a singularity point at which we'll live forever and even concepts such as living in simulations, for which we could decide upon our own height.

But even without such technological advancements, size should increase as per Cope's rule, and this should coincide with increasing longevity as per The Rate of Living Theory.

In the meantime though, lessened longevity, as with increased musculoskeletal injuries, could be a disadvantage had by people of tall stature, particularly those of extreme tall stature. Disadvantages such as these become social issues and thus I discuss them as such in the next chapter.

SOCIETY

A person's legs should be: "Long enough to reach the ground."

—6'4" Abraham Lincoln

Society is well aware of the advantages of tall stature, so much so that the challenges are overshadowed. And in parallel to this, we're criticized for our higher earning potential and increased usage of the planet's resources. These warrant a rebuttal.

One of the challenges we face is ill-fitting manufactured objects. Society can assist by changing regulations. I discuss this in this chapter, including for those horrendous airplane seats.

Tall women face some additional social issues, mostly relating to an expectation that women be shorter than men. For what my male perspective is worth, I discuss this predicament while presenting some positive and helpful notions. This is followed by a few points on bringing new tall life into this world.

Impression of Tall Stature

When I first decided I wanted to write this book, I did some digging to see what other people had written about tall stature. I came across a lot of books with the word 'tall' in the title. In particular, there have to be dozens, maybe even a hundred titles with the phrase 'standing tall'. The crazy thing is that none of these books have anything to do with tall stature. What they have in common, though, is how they use the word tall as a metaphor for competent, brave, proud, leader, and more generally, good.

Other phrases that are used similarly include, great stature, tall order, and tall, dark, and handsome. These are coherent with bigger is better, up is better, and many other similar metaphors.

It's clear that these metaphors demonstrate our positive impression of increased size and tall stature. Additionally, it has been recognized that metaphors are a crucial part of our understanding and thus they in turn influence our impressions.[105] This creates a positive feedback cycle that spirals our impression of tall stature increasingly 'upwards'.

Our preference for increased height is also apparent in the objects we create. Skyscrapers are a prime example here, where cities and nations are constantly 'one-upping' each other for the claim to the highest tower, free standing or otherwise. But this preference for larger objects is also present in more subtle ways. For instance, people have been found to overestimate the physical size of objects that have a high monetary value, such as a valuable coin or a face card.[106]

Positive sentiments for tall stature go far back into our past. For example, Egyptian wall paintings depict higher status people with greater stature and anthropologists uncovering prehistoric tombs find that the elegant crypts are mostly reserved for those of tall stature.[106]

In some cases, preference for tall stature is taken to the point of obsession, such as in King Frederick William's army of tall men known as the Potsdam Giants. William recruited soldiers, ranging from 6'2" to 7'2" in height, from all over Europe, resorting to forced breeding and kidnapping where necessary. Perhaps this was a form of fetishizing, something tall women are more commonly subject to.[51]

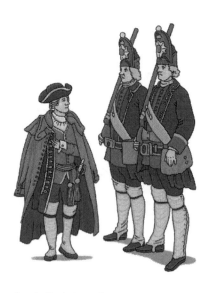

Preferences for tall stature have not gone unnoticed. Privilege calculators, of which there are a recent proliferation of, factor in tall stature as a positive. On a more scholarly note, the *American Sociological Association* writes, "American society is a society with a heightist premise: To be tall is to be good and to be short is to be stigmatized".[106]

Perhaps the most prominent and controversial measure of society's value of tall stature is success in the workplace. Taller people are more likely to hold positions of power such as CEOs who average over 6' tall and even US presidents who, more than three quarters of the time, are the taller of the two candidates. Taller people also tend to earn more. One study reported this increase to be about $166,000 over a thirty year career for a 6' person over a 5'5" person

($790 a year per inch).[107] Interestingly, height proved to account for the majority of the gender income gap.

While the greater earning capacity for increased height could once be explained by a greater ability to do physical work, this is no longer the case.[108] Instead, a variety of alternative theories have been proposed, ranging from a height bias to greater intelligence to various social relationships.[99,106,107,109-112] While on this topic, it's interesting to note that we tall people are more likely to strike out on our own and succeed as entrepreneurs, where ability is more greatly rewarded.[113]

In addition to greater earning capacity, some have tried to explain for preferential treatment of tall stature in general. The most common explanation is that it's due to a kind of primal remnant of our evolution.[99,109] The preference for tall stature has also been suggested to be related to an over-selection by women, a kind of mistake.[114] If one were to counter such negative sentiments, perhaps an effective tactic would be to say that preference for tall stature is more likely due to an innate understanding that evolution trends upwards, as it has since the dawn of life on our planet, starting from tiny single celled organisms.

Regardless of why, it's clear that tall stature is regarded positively in our culture. It's perhaps for this reason that people feel it's OK to ask us just how tall we are, exclaim at this height, and even make jokes about it. This, of course, isn't the case for other extreme variants such as short stature or a fat build. Even a thin build, which is often regarded positively, is unlikely to be remarked upon by a stranger in a grocery store as is the case for tall stature.

The most memorable comment I've received was from a little old man while I was feeling awkwardly tall on a subway in Hong Kong. He stared at me wide eyed for a good five minutes before finally popping the question.

What such commenters don't realize is that tall stature, being an extreme variant, isn't all hoops and glory and such comments grow tiresome. Hence, we would do well to arm ourselves with some clever retorts. A classy example was that of 6'4" Abraham Lincoln who responded with, after being asked how long a man's legs should be, "Long enough to reach the ground". A less classy example was that by 7'1" Wilt Chamberlin who, upon being asked how the weather was up there, proceeded to spit downwards and say, "It's raining." Many such retorts can be found on the web. For example, some tall people have taken to handing out a business card answering all the common questions. I plan to do this but with a card referring them to this book. Another helpful strategy is redirection. For example, the accompaniment of a cute or peculiar looking puppy will effectively switch the height related questions to: "What kind of a dog is that?" Curiously, eventually this question becomes similarly irksome, at least in my opinion.

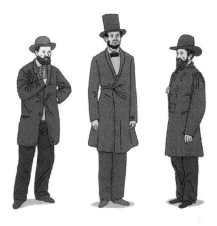

A classic comment people make is about playing basketball. We do have an advantage, so it would follow that we're more likely to play basketball than average height people, and at a 'higher' level. The more interesting question then is, how much more likely are we to play basketball? This isn't an easy question to answer, though a writer for Sports Illustrated attempted to by looking at height in the NBA and some extrapolated height stats from the *Centers for Disease Control*.[115] The finding was that, if you're an American between the heights of 6'6" and 6'8", you only have a 0.07 percent chance of being in the NBA. However, if you're 7' or taller, you have a whopping seventeen percent chance. However, the accuracy of this conclusion does come into question when you consider that height isn't perfectly normally distributed, and thus extrapolation will introduce error. Nevertheless, the chance is probably still whopping.

Another assumption people commonly make is that tall children are much older than they actually are. While some youngsters may appreciate this for gaining admission into otherwise restricted films and the like, it can also have the effect of losing out on some childhood. Also problematic can be the assumption of strength when in fact relative strength is diminished and injuries are more common, same as the assumption of competent leadership, which isn't always correct.

The lack of knowledge about tall stature isn't restricted to the general population, but also to professionals who find themselves working with us and even in the literature relating to variations in height. Firstly, there's a bizarre resistance to the notion that the taller body presents with altered fundamental characteristics that go far beyond a simply accentuated vertical extent. Additionally, the concept of an inverted U-shaped curve is poorly understood and seldom related. For example, while it's often said that tall men are the most successful dating population, it's not well known that success actually begins to decline in the extremes of height. In other words, women can actually find men to be **too** tall. Something similar can probably be said for earning capacity, cardiovascular disease, reproductive success, and happiness.

Another issue is the mistreatment that comes from being different, particularly during childhood. Anecdotally, as you read books on some tall people such as 6'11" Bill Walker,[116] there are many accounts of being bullied simply because of their height, particularly by short, aggressive males. And tall people are discouraged from fighting back because of our size advantage. Bill Walker attributes shorter male aggression to what is known as the Napoleon complex. Coincidently or not, it was Napoleon who eventually put an end to the Potsdam Giants battalion.

All this isn't to 'undermine' the struggles had by those of short stature. To begin with, society demonstrates quite the opposite opinion via metaphors: Fell short, shortcoming, short-sighted, talk down to, stoop low, belittle, etc. Increasing this negative sentiment of short stature is that it's known to coincide with famines, diseases, and a lack of prosperity. More generally, all the advantages associated with tall stature tend to be disadvantages for those of short stature.

But, a primary difference between short and tall stature in society is that the disadvantages of short stature are well recognized. For example, there are such prominent societies as *Little People of America* lobbying for their rights. Also, the use of the word heightism, as coined by the sociologist Saul Feldman,[117] is usually reserved for short people. And, while there's some research relating specifically to tall stature, there's far more relating to short stature. On a less essential level, sports where tall stature is an advantage often have weight classes, such as in weight lifting and fighting varieties, yet in sports where short stature is an advantage, such as in gymnastics and horse jockeying, there are no such compensations.

Perhaps a greater recognition of the struggles associated with short stature is justified, as the peak of the inverted U-shaped curve for height in modern society likely falls somewhere above average. Regardless, whether tall people or short people have it better seems to be a question researchers and the media are all too eager to answer. But while attempting to answer this question, they miss the elephant in the room; people near average height are above and beyond the most fortunate population. Firstly, they're favored by the natural world; if they weren't, the average height of the human race would have shifted. This translates to better resistance to injury and disease. Secondly, they're favored by the artificial world, due to the economy of scale that corresponds with catering to average size. What is needed then, for both short and tall people, are regulations to level the playing field.

Regulations and Disabilities

Companies, like humans, have evolved via a kind of selection, where the more fit survive and the lesser perish. Hence, companies that are successful also tend to be those that have harnessed the economies that come with scale. Unfortunately, this results in the neglect of outlier populations. Thus society must step in if equal accommodation of all people is to be achieved, which does appear to be our ambition. And in fact we do have regulations for this purpose. These are most often for the deaf, blind, wheelchair-bound, and obese. Most people would scoff to hear tall stature listed with these, and in most contexts they would be right to do so; tall stature coincides with extraordinary benefits while the popularly known issues are merely inconveniences, like poorly fitting clothing. However, with some less popularly known issues, such as the increased risk of injuries in car accidents and the ill-suited operating rooms and procedures for repairing these, you start to see that tall stature does in fact warrant additional regulations.

Admittedly, there are some regulations that do help. Automotive regulations, for example, often require certain aspects of cars be designed to accommodate from the fifth percentile female through to the ninety-fifth percentile male.

But in my humble opinion, leaving out five percent of the population is not acceptable, especially when we're dedicating massive amounts of resources to far less critical aspects of cars: Automated parallel parking versus sufficient space for the tall person to maintain a neutral spine posture. This becomes particularly infuriating when the effort and expense required to accommodate the upper percentiles is small in comparison to the potential benefit, such as adding an extra inch to head rest rails in order to reduce the high prevalence of whiplash injuries to which we're subject. The same goes for the extra few ounces of steel for seat rails required to increase legroom which would reduce the high prevalence of leg injuries experienced by us.

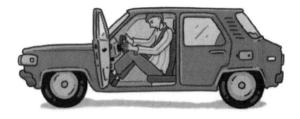

The most controversial ergonomics issue for us pertains to airplane seat legroom. For airlines, closer and thus more numerous seats leads to increased revenue. However, this translates to less legroom. This affects tall people most and can cause discomfort, joint pain, kneecap injuries, difficulty exiting the plane in an emergency, and even increased likelihood of deep vein thrombosis and pulmonary embolisms (blood clots can travel to the lungs, which is potentially lethal). Infuriatingly, these issues are becoming worse as airlines continue to shrink legroom while people continue to get taller. Seat pitch, the distance from the front of one seat to the back of the next, has dropped from thirty-five inches to thirty-one inches since the

1970s. A recent bill was supposed to put a stop to this insanity,[118] but was voted down.

Before venturing further into this issue, I have a concession to make—I haven't flown ever since my back first got bad about eight years ago. Being cramped in a tiny airplane seat with chronic back pain is my idea of a dreadful nightmare. I imagine I'll start flying again sometime soon given my back has mostly recovered, but I don't look forward to it. Now, with that concession out of the way, I'll move on to some potential solutions.

There's a device known as the Knee Defender which can provide some degree of relief by preventing the reclining of the seat in front. However, it has been banned by some airlines as it's notorious for causing arguments and has even led to fights. A recent patent application presents a more promising solution where seat rows can be adjusted fore and aft depending on the size of passengers in the rows.[119] This combined with assigned seating could solve the problem. However, it's likely shorter people would complain at losing space for which they paid equally. Furthermore, such additional hardware would increase weight and cost and thus it's unlikely to see widespread adoption.

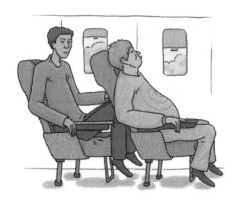

The simplest solution is to reserve an emergency exit or bulkhead seat. Sometimes it's possible to do so on booking websites, for a fee. Other times these vaunted seats may come by way of a sympathy upgrade, perhaps after having asked nicely at the desk. But this is the kind of thing that should be guaranteed, not merely hoped for nor paid for. It's this that the *Silicon Valley Tall Club* petitioned the *Department of Transportation* for, in addition to suing multiple airlines.[120] Unfortunately, the lawsuits were unsuccessful and petition dismissed on the grounds that such rule changes would be too costly for the airlines to implement and wouldn't be fair to other passengers.

Unlike tall people, obese people are often granted the additional space they require. This comes by way of a second seat. The *Canada Transportation Agency*, for instance, has a policy referred to as, "One person, one fare". In it, people considered disabled by obesity are granted a second seat at no extra charge. I find this puzzling, to put it gently, as we're afforded no such accommodation. Perhaps this problem could be solved if it could be proven that tall stature is a disability in this scenario.

This raises the question of exactly what is a disability. The *World Health Organization* explains that the term disability covers "activity limitations, and participation restrictions".[121] Perhaps it could be demonstrated that extremely tall people at times may avoid flying simply due to the discomfort that comes from being tall in tiny airplane seats. Then tall stature could gain acceptance as a disability in this scenario, making it straight forward to grant extra space one way or another. The question of who should pay for the additional legroom is relevant to the section to come.

Taxation

The purpose of taxation is to provide funds for achieving the common goals of a population. It's often debated how these taxes should be applied. Under optimal taxation theory, the aim is to tax ability and not effort, thereby avoiding the discouragement of effort. However, it's difficult to separate these and simpler to tax earnings while accounting for the more obvious liabilities such as children, being a single parent, personal disabilities, mortgage interest payments, charitable contributions, and health expenditures.

However, with modern population studies it's now possible to determine what abilities, and the characteristics which correlate with these, increase earning potential. And as pointed out by Harvard business economist and former Bush administration advisor Gregory Mankiw, height is such a characteristic and thus tall people should be taxed at higher rates.[122]

A counter argument Conor Clark, a writer for the Atlantic, made is that models without exceptions are rare. The comparison he used was the inconsistency in moral decisions for the greater good; while it may seem intuitively obvious to reroute a runaway train to a smaller population to reduce casualties, this same moral logic isn't so obvious when it comes to harvesting one person's organs to save many. Similarly, intuition tells us that we shouldn't tax people simply for their height.

While this counter argument is somewhat convincing, there's a stronger one, and that's that taller peoples' increased cost of living works to offset our greater earning potential. Food is the obvious contributor here. While at first this may seem like a relatively small expenditure compared to how much more we tend to earn, consider that we have taller children who will also require more food. Additionally, in less prosperous times and in rationing situations, quantity of food becomes much more critical. Another source for a higher cost of living is increased medical expenditures.

A less obvious one is increased cost of clothing and other manufactured objects; though these may be priced the same on shelves, we more often must buy new and sometimes specialty or even custom items. There are all kinds off hidden extras to our cost of living. And even when we're done living, our estates may be dinged with extra-large coffin and excavation fees,[123] assuming you go that route.

So while the increase in earnings tapers off with height, the costs ramp up. These combine to form an upside-down U-shaped curve, where there's a height at which financial situations begin to worsen. Determining the height at which this occurs would be a complex endeavor, and one that's outside the scope of this book. Though if such an endeavor were undertaken, and the peak of the curve was found to be in the tall range, there's yet one more point to be raised.

As I discussed in the previous chapter, there's some evidence that we tend to die younger. Thus, if this is true and if we're to enjoy the same number of retirement years, then we must earn more. When you consider this, it's likely that the math would show that we should be taxed at a lower rate. Furthermore, we should get seniors' discounts at a younger age. Bring on the free coffee!

Environmental Implications

Our higher earning capacity and higher cost of living may have a balancing effect overall when it comes to social equality. But as far as the environment is concerned, at a first glance it would appear that our net effect is a greater toll. We require more food and water, more energy for transportation, and larger manufactured objects. As the world becomes ever more populated, resources wane, and pollution proliferates, tall stature has the appearance of being a disadvantage to the human race.

This gives rise to the notion that humanity would benefit if the average height were reduced rather than increased as is the current trend. There are many proponents to this notion with a variety of ideas for how it could be carried out, including revised nutrition guidelines and genetic modification. An entire website, entitled *The Incredible Shrinking Man*, revolves around the idea of shrinking humans to a height of 1'8". Perhaps the greatest proponent, though, is Thomas Samaras of *Reventropy Associates*. His forty years of research, all of which hinges around a height reduction proposal, represents a formidable contribution towards the understanding of human height.

Samaras points out that absolute physical strength, which correlates with height, was advantageous to early humans for hunting, fighting, and survival, and benefitted men in particular, permitting them first choice of food and mates.[99] Yet in modern times, Samaras continues, knowledge, intellect, communication ability, social skills, and creativity are what matter. And though taller people tend to be more intelligent and hold positions of greater power, Samaras strives to prove that this is permitted merely by humanity's unfounded bias and prejudice for greater height.

On the other hand, Samaras sees two great disadvantages of taller stature which justify the shrinking proposal. The first is the aforementioned environmental ramifications. The second is that shorter people, by his research and assuming socioeconomic status is controlled for, tend to live longer. Ironically, his second insight detracts from his own argument; by living longer, the shorter person increases their lifetime toll on the planet. Furthermore, the environmental load of tall people decreases in step with our lower reproductive success.

This of course is all in the short term. In the long term, a taller species would in theory live longer as per the Rate of Living Theory. Another potential benefit would be greater intelligence via bigger brains. In general, there evidently must be considerable benefits to increased size as evolution trends upwards as per Cope's rule. Certainly there are challenges, as demonstrated by the Lilliput Effect, but to ignore the long term benefits of increased size is shortsighted.

One thing the shrinking proposal would achieve is to increase the number of people that can simultaneously live on the planet. If this is what society seeks, then perhaps the proposal has some merit. However, like with levying us with greater taxes, there's a kind of intuitive feeling that the proposed social engineering is a faulty path, as is the same for the intentional increasing of height via genetic muddling or otherwise. Perhaps this is because these seem related to the many stereotypes and prejudices that modern society seeks to abolish.

In actuality, there are issues to be addressed that present far more certain, effective, and unbiased ways to decrease our environmental toll on the planet. For instance, people worldwide throw out nearly half of all food produced,[124] a lot of which is meat, a most energy exhaustive food source. Those in the developed world are particularly at fault given they consume more than ten times the resources per capita compared to those in developing countries.[125] Furthermore, people are unscrupulous with water usage, spew astounding amounts of carbon into the atmosphere despite the availability of renewables, and design products with intentionally short life cycles, the list goes on.

All of this being said, it still weighs particularly heavily on us to abide by environmentally friendly practices as, on a daily basis, we have a greater impact on the environment. Furthermore, society looks to tall people for leadership, thereby providing us an opportunity to set an example.

The Tall Female Predicament

As a tall man, I can't possibly relate to some of the struggles tall women experience. Nevertheless, I'm confident I've summarized some of the literature in such a way that it's both interesting and, later in the section, helpful. But I'll start with an anecdote of my own.

There was a lot of buzz when *My Giant Life*, a reality show about tall women, aired. So Huffington Post jumped on the opportunity to interview two of the stars, 6'6" Colleen Smith and 6'9" Lindsay Hayward. And to keep things interesting, they decided to video conference in a tall guy as a guest. That guy was me.

Prior to the show, I was told to prepare several questions to ask. So you can understand why I was taken off-guard when the host turned it around and asked me a rather loaded question. She wanted to know my girlfriend's height. 5'8", I replied. The inevitable guffaw about tall guys and much shorter girls ensued. My follow-up was that this isn't because I have a preference for much shorter women, but rather that there are simply more near-average fish in the sea (5'8" is actually kinda tall, though relatively speaking here). On a side note, I hope this metaphor didn't offend my girlfriend's mother who happened to be watching the shenanigans.

A speed dating study backs me up on this matter, finding that men aren't all that selective for height.[126] Instead of height, we tend to be more selective for signs of fertility, like youth and proportions, characteristics that don't correlate all that tightly with height. Furthermore, we're less selective in general. This is due to Bateman's principle, where males, given far more numerous sperm than females have eggs, better increase our chances of reproductive success via multiple partners rather than selectivity. What's more, females are at greater risk from a sub-par coupling given they must bear the child and, historically, play a larger role in raising the child. Because of all this, females tend to be more selective than males. This disparity is evidently highest for tall men, given their tendency to have more life partners and greater rates of divorce.[127]

Women's selectivity, on the other hand, comes in the form of a preference for significantly taller men. This is about ten inches as per the same speed dating study. The somewhat wearisome explanation for this, as per evolutionary psychology, is that throughout the majority of human evolution, male strength was crucial for hunting and providing protection, and strength increases with height.

What all this translates to is that tall men are statistically at an advantage in finding a partner while tall women are not. Tall women's harder time finding a partner is one possible explanation for lower reproductive success, the other being, as for tall men, a greater prevalence of health issues.[128]

Whether we like it or not, men and women are both products of evolution, and these mechanisms are deeply engrained within human genetics. That being said, there's a magnifying social component that's only recently beginning to diminish. Society has imposed gender roles where men have been expected to be the primary bread winners and females to stay home and bear and take care of children. While height is favorable in the workplace for both leadership[129] and earning ability,[110] it does not confer the same benefits in the traditional female role. In fact, shorter women were preferred as they were expected to submit to male dominance. And because worth was judged in these respective roles, society preferred taller men and shorter women. The media further reinforces society's view on gender and height by depicting male heroes as significantly taller than females, even using props and trick photography where necessary to achieve this.

A consequence of all this was that it became common sentiment that tall women were at risk of depression. This is what gave rise to the proliferation of height reduction treatments in women, which ironically led to fertility issues.[76] Other justifications for height reduction treatments included difficulty finding clothes[130] and a tendency towards slouching,[80] which is harmful to the spine.

But as we move into the twenty-first century, a marked decrease in society's preference for short women is taking place. This has been pushed along by the gradual transition towards workplace gender neutrality. Like men, women's value in the workplace has been found to benefit from increased stature.[129]

Additionally, new prestigious roles have arisen which confer advantages to tall women, examples being in modeling and athletics. With this transition has come an appreciation for women outside of the traditional family setting. Similarly, it's becoming more acceptable for males to stay home and raise children, thereby placing less emphasis on traditional concepts of masculinity, and thus height, in measuring the value of a man.

The evolving structure of society in general has diminished gender roles. Military and police forces now provide protection, social systems provide for the unemployed, benefits packages support women with maternity leave, and government agencies work towards ensuring equal earning opportunities. More women in the workplace, where tall stature receives preferential treatment, has led to tall women gaining greater acceptance.

Another helpful facet of the twenty-first century is the rise of social media, which has connected similar groups of people, such as the tall female minority population, across the globe. Being able to find others to share similar experiences with, relate to, and support is most beneficial, #TallGirlProblems. That which gave rise to social media, the World Wide Web, has also been instrumental in providing access to tall female consumers, leading to a rise in availability of clothing specifically for tall women.

The tall female predicament is rapidly improving. The greatest testament to this is the decreased usage of, and increased threshold for, height reduction treatments. While in the 1950s women were treated at as low as 5'8",[80] this is now typically above 6'. Another helpful notion for tall girls is that dating preferences for both genders opens up with age, thereby expanding the potential dating pool for tall women. This parallels the modern tall woman's experience with her height in general; she struggles with it through adolescence yet comes to accept, and what's more, appreciate it as an adult where tall stature confers extensive social benefits.[51,131]

Nevertheless, tall women, particularly extremely tall women, continue to be at a statistical disadvantage when it comes to finding a partner. In light of this, I mention the following helpful insights.

As already stated, it isn't because tall men prefer average height women that we tend to end up with them. Rather, it's due to probabilities. So, rather than becoming discouraged when seeing average height women with tall men, tall women are best served by using this to reinforce an understanding that dating is a probabilities game.

Being open to partnering with a shorter man is the single best way to increase probabilities. This has some other added benefits too. To begin with, it makes it possible to be selective for qualities that are more important in the modern world, including similar interests, personality, intelligence, humor, and job. Additionally, by finding a partner that's OK with a taller woman, a man more secure with his masculinity is ensured while the less secure are automatically weeded out. I'd also like to point out that a taller woman who partners with a shorter man would be more likely to bring a closer to average height girl into the world who might avoid some of the same struggles. Then again, by that point in life, the tall woman may appreciate her height so much that this is a moot point. This runs parallel to the finding that, while a taller man does make a woman initially more happy, this gradually weakens with time, totally dissipating by eighteen years.[132]

All this being said, the instinct for a taller male is strong, and some women will prefer other approaches for increasing probabilities, of which there are many. For example, probabilities can also be boosted by living in large cities. Online dating, despite its many pitfalls, does similarly. There are some dating sites that revolve around tall women. As much as this may at first seem ideal, outcomes are prone to being of the superficial tall girl fetish variety. Rather, it's better if height limits are placed on both genders, despite how this may decrease the numbers. Rather humorously, one tall dating site claims to do this, but by using limits of 6' for men yet only 5'5" for women. You'd be right if you guessed the site was started by a man. The tall community expressed outrage over this. The result was that the founder said he'd change the limit, though he has yet to do so.

Probabilities can also be boosted by seeking out tall populations. This might at first appear to be a suggestion to move to the Netherlands where average male height is 6'1". But as helpful as that would be, it isn't likely feasible. Rather, what I mean by tall populations is groups where tall people tend to congregate. These are primarily related to sports which confer advantages to tall stature, including basketball, volleyball, and swimming. In addition to probabilities, sports, when played well, boost confidence which in turn helps in attracting a partner. Furthermore, these sports give a sense of purpose to height, helping the tall female come to embrace it.[133]

Sports are also a source for finding tall female role models, such as 6'8" WNBA star Britney Grinner as demonstrated by her book, *In My Skin*. Other helpful literature written by tall women include *The Tall Book* by Arianne Cohen and the dissertation entitled, *Should women fear being too tall? A study examining the experiences of very tall women.*[131] More research is also currently underway by Julie Booth of Coventry University in the UK (her work relates to very tall young adults in general). On a less academic note, there are also the many blogs written by tall women.

New Tall Life

As contraceptives, abortions, modern medicine, and sex education become more readily available, the most biologically fulfilling act of having children has become a conscious decision with tremendous and complex moral and ethical implications. This decision is being demonstrated by educated people who are, for whatever reason, less often making the choice to have children.[134] A complete discussion on this topic requires a scope that's far beyond that of this book. Nevertheless, the context of this book warrants mention of the following insights.

Three and a half billion years of evolution on this planet has led to you. Each and every one of your ancestors has reproduced, continuing the chain in a most momentous single elimination tournament which, if you follow the footsteps, has the potential to be extended indefinitely. Your very own improbable existence is a testament to your ancestors' determination to propagate, a determination you have almost certainly inherited.

Yet, despite such will, the vast majority of species, more than ninety-nine times as many as are currently alive today, have gone extinct. It's natural selection which presides over this judgement, while it's adaptation via genetic variations that paved the way to the formation and survival of the remaining species, including our own. The probability of any one variation being preferential in the eyes of natural selection is slim, though a sufficient quantity of variations is generated such that some are.

As I explained in the first chapter and expanded upon numerous times throughout this book, increased height, in its most profound sense, represents such a genetic variation upon which natural selection may act. It confers both considerable advantages and disadvantages. Most importantly, the taller body is relatively weaker but absolutely stronger and requires more energy in the absolute sense but less in the relative sense, leading to a slower rate of living. The question is whether the pros outweigh the cons. In the long run, they do, as is postulated by Cope's rule. Yet this is in the long term, meaning increases occur most gradually. Tall stature, on the other hand, corresponds with a rapid increase in height. The consequence of this is some health issues, namely increased risk of musculoskeletal injuries and cancer. And in the very long term, the laws of scaling place a cap on maximum size and mass extinctions are less kind to larger species, as per the Lilliput Effect.

Yet perhaps we've begun evolving on our own terms via technological and cultural adaptation. This new form of evolution has a tendency to mirror natural evolution, where only the fittest prosper. This is exemplified by companies catering, because of the economies that come with scale, to the average size while neglecting the outliers such as tall people and thereby creating ergonomic and other health hazards. But of course there are far more heinous examples like abysmal wealth distribution, discrimination, and unspeakable atrocities.

In parallel to this though, we see cultural and technological advancements being used for good. Gradually, levels of accommodation are being raised for people of all shapes and sizes. And even more encouraging are advancements that include technological breakthroughs, regulations, programs, charities, and activism for preserving the environment, peace, human rights, equality, and health and wellbeing of all people in general. These are movements one would be hard pressed to explain the source for in the context of evolution via natural selection.

In essence, our ability to adapt via cultural and technological advancement has presented us with a choice: Do we carry on a path as or more callous than that grooved by natural selection, or do we break new ground, and see to it that every person is ensured a basic level of wellbeing while simultaneously side stepping the next mass extinction? If you believe humanity's choices tilt toward the latter, a belief that surely must be paralleled by your own choices, then you'll likely also believe that it's worth bringing new life into this world, no matter how tall, short, or otherwise different.

AFTERWARD

Being extremely tall (6'7", 99.97th percentile, +3.5 standard deviations) has had an enormous impact on my life. Of course as my younger self, with limited experiences and knowing no alternative, I was oblivious of this. Further, I knew little about the implications of tall stature. Had I, this would have undoubtedly proven most helpful in the challenging years that were to come. I wish I could go back and educate my younger self on tall stature. This, clearly, isn't possible. But what I can do, and hope to have done with this book, is to help those on route to tall stature such as I once was myself. And now, to complete this book, I give a brief account of the life events that led up to its writing.

My own tall tale made a clever use of foreshadowing. At 16, my height was certainly a factor in both making my regional volleyball team, and the resulting back injury after a weeklong intense training camp. But my youthful spine appeared to forgive me, and sadly, I forgot. As the years went by, I had many other injuries. Yet I ploughed on through, much as is expected by our sporting culture, as I greatly enjoyed the advantages my height conferred.

My height opened many doors for me. The trick though, was not knocking my noggin on the way through. For example, I made my high school basketball team despite my total lack of experience and coordination— but then the foolish coach left me riding the pine all season. The volleyball coach, on the other hand, gave me some court time, and this paid off as I eventually became his most valuable player.

Excelling at volleyball gave a kind of purpose to my height, built up my confidence, and was incredibly beneficial in the social sense. It made it OK to be different. Though this isn't to say I didn't have those awkward moments as I tried to 'fit in'. A most memorable one was when my high school prom date requested I dance with either just my legs or just my arms, as both were clearly too much for me to handle. Less memorable examples are all the height related comments, as there have been so many that they have blurred together. Yet, annoyances such as these mattered little next to the benefits my height provided me in sports.

But these benefits came at a price. It was my second year on the provincial volleyball team when my gradually worsening knee injury forced me to step back from the sport, forgoing what had otherwise looked to be a promising varsity run. A physiotherapist figured it was jumper's knee (patella femoral syndrome), an injury tall people are at increased risk of, and an MRI turned up a partial patella tendon tear. After I eased up on it, however, my knee got to the point where I could play in recreational leagues as I coached on the side.

I also took another crack at basketball but found it was just as hard on my body, particularly for wrecking my ankle. Then I took up squash thinking it must be more gentle since you see so many older people playing, including my seventy year old varsity coach who could whip my butt. Boy, was I wrong. So then I tried swimming. How can water hurt you, right? I tore my rotator cuff. But all of these injuries were minor compared to the one that put my life on hold.

It was the foreshadowed back injury. An MRI of my spine, which made my heart sink while shattering my youthful sense of invincibility, showed much desiccation, multiple disc protrusions, end plate fractures, end plate osteophytes, and a Schmorl's node. So ensued my multi-year adventure into our medical system. More tests were ordered including a bone scan, more MRIs, blood work, and many x-rays including for a leg length discrepancy check which rather comically required two x-ray films to capture the whole of my leg. And armed with this data I saw doctors, physiotherapists, an osteopath, a chiropractor, massage therapists, a physiatrist, an orthotist, surgeons, and even a spine researcher. Over countless appointments, there were biomechanical assessments, the prescribing of exercises, spine cracking, various kinds of electrical shocks, ultrasounds, infrared, traction, massaging, even of my feet, many back braces including a custom molded one, acupuncture, and many drugs. Most of these did not help, though some did.

Of all the help I got, the most beneficial was that by Stuart McGill, the world renowned spine researcher whom my stepfather most helpfully arranged an introduction to. This came by way of a few consultations as well as studying his books. His emphases on neutral spine posture and removing the cause were of immeasurable value to me. McGill also told me these things take time to heal, that I'd be better in a couple years, and to be patient. But patient I was not. This, I'm certain, made matters worse.

To say that my back injury dominated my life just doesn't do it justice. For starters, I had to give up all the sports I enjoyed. But even just sitting became a problem, which meant I had to give up such simple things as playing music, going to the movies, and taking road trips. It put my life on hold to the point where I lost many of my friends, my relationship was affected, and I was left struggling to figure out how I'd earn a living. The fact that back pain is invisible worsens matters as well as the expectations of strength that come with being a tall man. My back pain also had an infuriating tendency to flare up at the worst possible times, namely when people were counting on me. For example, long hours at my hospitalized father's side triggered an incapacitating set of back spasms, leaving me bedridden for an entire week, one of the few weeks he had left.

It was for situations such as this that I worked so hard towards improving my back. I did this with what is commonly referred to as conservative treatment as I explain below. I did consider surgery, but because of the challenges of operating on the thoracic spine, I was told I wasn't a candidate. In hindsight, I see this as a blessing in disguise; even if surgery had been successful, I wouldn't have learned how to deal with it myself, and events likely would have repeated themselves.

Of all the approaches I took in improving my back, there are five that I think stand out. The first is a variety of exercise for improving stability and correcting posture. Admittedly, I had a hard time keeping at these on my own, and that's where my yoga practice came in. The many positive aspects, including the sense of community and the focus on the mind in addition to the body, helped to keep me coming back. And, while there are many yoga poses I feel were bad for my injury, I was able to modify these. I've been practicing yoga for nearly seven years now and hope to continue practicing for many years to come. Yoga in particular I think is responsible for my more than one inch increase in stature as my back was recovering. I was so alarmed at this increase that I asked my family doctor if he thought there was any chance I was still growing despite being in my mid-twenties. He assured me there was not.

The second approach was endurance exercise via the low impact sport of cycling, the one sport that became a kind of compensation for me for the others I'd had to give up. I didn't need anyone to tell me I felt better after intense endurance exercise; it was quite clear to me that it both decreased my pain and elevated my mood. And while I'd tried narcotics to help me with my pain, I greatly preferred the natural high and pain relief which are thought to come from endocannabinoids and endorphins. Sadly, I wasn't aware of a geometrical irregularity of my hip joint called femoral acetabular impingement (FAI) where flexion is restricted, and the repeated flexion with cycling led to a hip labral tear. Ironically, if I'd used standard length pedal cranks instead of extra-long cranks that were proportional to my height, I don't think this would have been such an issue. I did consult a surgeon, perhaps the best here in Canada. He said he'd probably have to send me to the US as I'm too tall for his setup! But the main deterrent for me is the long recovery time, some six months. Besides, I'm back to the point where I can ride casually now. As far as cardio, I get this from an elliptical or brisk walk instead.

And I do mean brisk. I've affectionately nicknamed my girlfriend Baby Steps for her struggle to keep up. This is because, at 5'8", she's nearly a foot shorter than me. This height gap came up in the Huffington Post interview I mentioned in the last chapter. My explanation was that there are simply more 5'8" fish in the sea and so I caught the best fish I could independent of size. And as I explained earlier, women are more selective for height, which might have contributed at least a bit initially in my ending up with such a wonderful partner. I still remember the moment we met. An old friend of mine, whom I saw eye to eye with (same height), and I decided on a whim to take a seat with two pretty ladies at a pub. After a pleasant chat, they accepted our challenge for a beach volleyball match the following day and the rest is history. The name of the pub was *Molly Bloom's*—and so became our puppy's name, Molly, who, with her four scurrying paws, has stepped in for Baby Steps as my new walking companion. Besides the cardiovascular benefits, walking is also therapeutic for back pain, helps to improve spine stability, and provides an opportunity to hone postural awareness.

Getting back on track here, the third approach was that of nutrition, and it was my mother who helped me most in this regard. Specifically, I began a mostly plant based diet, though with lots of fish high in omega-3s given their role in reducing inflammation. Such a diet, as I mentioned in chapter seven, Longevity, is also thought to reduce the risk of cancer. This is particularly important for tall people given our elevated risk. My new diet was a huge step up from the highly processed packaged meats and frozen pizzas I was relying on in my university years. A tricky thing with diet though is that feedback can be slow, and this does make it hard at times to keep it up. A factor that does help is an ergonomically suitable kitchen to work in.

While on the topic of food, it's interesting to point out that, as a kid, I consumed a lot of cow's milk on a daily basis. This may have been a contributing factor towards my final adult stature being more than half a foot taller than what would have been predicted by averaging my parents' heights (5'6" and 6') and adjusting for gender. However, I do have some tall relatives outside my immediate family, and it was noted that I was a rather 'long' baby, suggesting that it was more genetics and perhaps early nutrition that led to my height. And in fact, my South African father passed down Dutch and German genes to me. So while I consider myself Canadian, it's no wonder why the girl in an Amsterdam pub was sure I was just a Dutchmen pretending to be Canadian as a pickup tactic. What can you do, eh?

The fourth approach I tried was mindfulness. I took meditation classes, studied various teachings including those of Jon Kabat-Zinn, emphasized mindfulness in my yoga practice, and began a regular sitting practice (for as long as my back would tolerate) as I tried to learn acceptance. Though I think mindfulness has incredible potential, particularly by separating pain from suffering, the necessary discipline is something I struggle with. My own acceptance I think arrived more from the simple passage of time. Perhaps if I'd learned mindfulness as a child, as I think should be standard practice in our education system, then I could've coped better.

The fifth and most helpful approach I took was adapting my ergonomics with the tall solutions I explained in chapter five, Ergonomics. I became meticulous about eliminating any potential sources for slouching. A couple of the more helpful solutions included the raised cutting board and the extended snow shovel. Perhaps the most helpful was adapting my Honda Element. I've since sat in some of the cars I used to drive, and it's now clear to me that these played a lead role in damaging my spine by forcing me to slouch. In addition to adaptations, another helpful project was my zero gravity workstation setup. This gave my back a chance to rest while I was still getting work done.

By a lucky coincidence, my education was relevant to my height and injury. Having gone through mechanical engineering, I'd had much opportunity to hone my skills at designing, building, and problem solving and this helped me in adapting my ergonomics. My graduate work was related to mass customization methods, which tall people in particular may benefit from, and biomechanics, which helped me understand why the mechanics of tall stature are so different. Despite these benefits, the stress of such prolonged education took its toll on me, and I think it only a slight coincidence that its completion occurred near the same time my back pain was subsiding.

Somewhere between the fourth and fifth years after that fateful MRI, my back pain had mostly disappeared. I still do experience crippling spasms now and then and there are the many other injuries that continue to cause me problems, but my more moderate and adaptive approach to life has allowed me to reclaim much of what I'd lost. I try hard not to take this for granted, yet inevitably I do at times.

Besides musculoskeletal injuries, another health issue I have had is a minor arrhythmia, more specifically a high number of palpitations known as pre ventricular contractions (PVCs). Traditionally, these aren't thought to be of concern. However, recent research is finding that PVCs are a precursor for atrial fibrillation. And given atrial fibrillation is of considerably higher risk for tall people in the first place, and interventions are poorly suited to taller patients, I don't think a high number of PVCs is something to be ignored. But I came to realize it was stress that was the trigger for me, and after getting through a particularly rough patch in my life, they began to subside.

Besides the health issues, another defining aspect of my life is my striving for independence. It's this which has given rise to a variety of entrepreneurial endeavors, of which the self-publishing of this book is the latest. My biggest endeavor though, revolves around custom footwear technology. It's fascinating to be in the business while disruptive technologies are on the verge of making custom affordable for both the masses and people with unusual shapes or sizes, like tall people. My own difficulties finding shoes has been exacerbated by a ginormous big toe. This extraordinary phalange skipped a generation, passed straight from my Grandpa to me. He struggled with it, particularly when trying to fit size fifteen feet into size twelve boots while in the U.S. navy. For me, this large toe was the source of yet another injury. I discovered the cracked sesamoid when I had an MRI of my foot done for the purposes of building a three dimensional simulation model of a human foot for my graduate work. With custom footwear though, I have essentially removed the cause, and I no longer have pain in the joint. Another population that appreciates optimal fitting footwear is diabetics, such as my own father who had to have his foot chopped off in his final days. Custom footwear probably wouldn't have made much of a difference for him, though would for many other diabetics given the risk of ulceration. Footwear is incredibly important, and we often take this for granted.

I was intrigued to learn that tall people in general are more likely to go down the entrepreneurial route. The researchers who discovered this attributed it to tall people tending to be more successful and thus feeling they would do better to strike off on their own. Perhaps this is true, but I also think growing up different creates a kind of independent nature. For me, this was amplified by inheriting my father's independent spirit, where he was happiest as a consulting engineer and was a most epic DIY enthusiast and jack of all trades.

A challenge with entrepreneurship is that it lacks the economy of scale, inherent efficiency as per the laws of scaling, and opportunity for specialization available to the larger entities with which it competes. The consequence is that you have to work much harder and/or smarter for equal gains. This of course is magnified by its being a new venture. The flip side, I believe, is that more creativity arises, and thus potential for advancement.

Impressed upon me while writing this book was the iterative nature of such a project. I now better appreciate what is meant by the expression, "Premature optimization is the root of all evil". The first draft of the book was twice the current length and filled with equations, and I unwisely polished it only to totally rewrite it. I made this mistake over and over again. I also changed the scope several times. I wanted to stay true to my purpose though I also wanted the book to be applicable to as many people as possible, two contradictory objectives. I considered expanding it to include short stature or maybe just making it about height in general. However, these would have driven me off course. In the end, what I recognized was that anyone who relates to or works with tall people should also find this book informative. This includes family and friends for starters, but more than that, professionals such as physicians, designers, teachers, researchers, and regulators. When you consider that each of us is thought to be a mere seven handshakes from anyone in the world, suddenly the audience for this book seems a fair bit larger. And beyond this, anyone with an interest in the various topics covered should appreciate the book given its unique perspective.

Of all the content in this book, I feel that the tall solutions are the most novel and the biggest contribution. It's tall men who will benefit most from these, given their greater share of pure vertical extent. For tall women, the greater issues are of a social nature, probably due to society's expectation that women be shorter than men. While I have tried to address these in the final chapter of this book, I'm certain that a tall female author could've done these greater justice. It's my hope that there will be a second edition of this book and the tall female predicament section will be expanded.

Beyond ergonomics and social issues though, perhaps the more concerning issue is increased cancer rates which adversely affect longevity. This was a most difficult issue to learn and write about, particularly because I have no personal experiences to draw on, for which I'm grateful, nor anything novel to contribute on the topic. Rather, the chapter is there merely to raise awareness and encourage taller people to make a particular effort to follow what is becoming common lifestyle advice including for diet and exercise. With this, perhaps the playing field will be leveled. Unlike others who address this topic, however, I delight in pointing out that larger species live longer, and thus taller people are paving the way for a longer living human species.

And now, at last, this book must come to an end. Yet the project does not end here. Rather, it's continued on www.Tall.Life, which is both a mirror and extension of the contents of this book. It's my intention that it will become a gathering place for discussions on tall stature and human height in general. I hope you'll join in and spread the word. It's my sincerest wish that this project will be helpful to the many tall people around the globe, but also outliers in general as we seek to accommodate people of all shapes, sizes, and other differences.

ACKNOWLEDGEMENTS

There are a great many people I'd like to thank for seeing me through to the end of this journey of a book.

To begin with, I'd like to thank my partner, Brandy Eberhardt. She is the one person whose support I could not have done without. Her patience, encouragement, ideas, and constructive criticism were most appreciated. I also thank William Abbott, a philosophy professor and my stepfather, for his support, inspiration, contributions, and generous teachings. Next I thank my mother, Christine Jewell, whose expertise as a research librarian and meticulousness as a linguist came in most handy. As a mother though, her words of wisdom, as I'd wager came from your mother too, provide a remarkably succinct substitute for the some 35,000 words of this book: Sit up straight and eat your vegetables! As for my father and engineer, Jasper Lochner, his creative and independent spirit is written all over this book. My Grandparents, Marilynn and Ken Jewell, a language professor and creative writer, also steered me on my path.

I'd also like to thank my various proof readers. My good friend Josh Moore made many critical suggestions, including to remove the naked Vitruvian man from the cover; this would have grossed out most potential readers! Another critical suggestion came from a long-time friend, Way Ngo, and that was to cut out about 20,000 words from the first two chapters. And my most astute pal Jason Gillham pointed out that I should be writing in the first person. All of these were absolutely essential.

I've also had a lot of help from the tall community. Dan Deceuster, the founder of a fantastic tall clothing brand, Tall Slim Tees, helped me make the tone of the book more inviting. Conan Stevens, the 7' actor from Game of Thrones, lent me his insights from movie making and encouraged me to simplify the book and add in more personal anecdotes to make it more relatable. Other community members who helped include, Terry Levering, Tim Hopper, and Julie Booth.

It was truly a stroke of good luck becoming acquainted with Julie Booth, an occupational therapist and senior lecturer at Coventry University in the UK. She is currently doing her PhD and it revolves around tall people! Her advancing of knowledge on tall stature is most needed. I give my thanks to Julie for her feedback and encouragement.

I also thank my illustrator, Taras Kharechko. At 6'7" himself, he really has an appreciation for tall predicaments and this comes out in his illustrations. My cover illustrator, Sumit Roy, also did a spectacular job.

I'd also like to extend my thanks to those that helped me get through my own back pain, including Professor Stuart McGill and the instructors at Moksha Yoga Waterloo, and those who were patient with me and continued to believe in me as I recovered, including my doctoral advisors Sanjeev Bedi and Jan Huissoon and business partner Tezera Ketema.

Finally, I thank you, the readers. For the tall among you, many of whom have and continue to contribute ideas for this project, it's our common ground for which I have found justification for writing this book. The project has given me a sense of purpose, an opportunity to be of use, a chance to learn for the betterment of my own life, and has brought meaning to my experiences with my height.

REFERENCES

1.	Anthropometric Reference Data for Children and Adults⊡: United States ,. *Centers Dis Control Provention*. 2010.

2.	Stewart JM, Clarke D. "Hes dizzy when he stands up": An introduction to initial orthostatic hypotension. *J Pediatr*. 2011;158(3).

3.	Arvedsen SK, Damgaard M, Norsk P. Body height and blood pressure regulation in humans during anti-orthostatic tilting. *Am J Physiol Regul Integr Comp Physiol*. 2012;302(8).

4.	Mitchell G, van Sittert SJ, Skinner JD. The structure and function of giraffe jugular vein valves. *South African J Wildl Res*. 2009;39(2).

5.	G. Mitchella JDS. How Giraffe Adapt to Their Extraordinary Shape. *Trans R Soc South Africa*. 1993;48(2).

6.	Macho GA1, Spears IR, Leakey MG, McColl DJ, Jiang Y, Abel R, Nakatsukasa M KY. An exploratory study on the combined effects of external and internal morphology on load dissipation in primate capitates: its potential for an understanding of the positional and locomotor repertoire of early hominins. *Folia Primatol*. 2010.

7.	Hone DWE, Benton MJ. The evolution of large size: how does Cope's Rule work? *Trends Ecol Evol*. 2005;20(1).

8.	Sekerak RJ, Zimmermann KP. Chin-up strength tests:

169

does stature matter? *J Sports Med Phys Fitness*. 2008;48(1).

9.   Robinson MR, Hemani G, Gomez CM-, Esko T, Shakhbazov K, Powell JE. Population genetic differentiation of height and body mass index across Europe.

10.   Burton RF. Why is the body mass index calculated as mass/height ^{2} , not as mass/height ^{3}? *Ann Hum Biol*. 2007;34(6).

11.   MacKay NJ. Scaling of human body mass with height: The body mass index revisited. *J Biomech*. 2010;43(4).

12.   Diverse T, Collaborative P, Mcgee DL. Weight-height relationships and body mass index: some observations from the Diverse Populations Collaboration. *Am J Phys Anthropol*. 2005;128(1).

13.   Taki Y, Hashizume H, Sassa Y, et al. Correlation among body height, intelligence, and brain gray matter volume in healthy children. *Neuroimage*. 2012;59(2).

14.   McDaniel M a. Big-brained people are smarter: A meta-analysis of the relationship between in vivo brain volume and intelligence. *Intelligence*. 2005;33(4).

15.   Stuart. *Back Mechanic: The Step-by-Step McGill Method to Fix Back Pain*. Gravenhurst: Backfitpro; 2015.

16.   Rivner MH, Swift TR, Crout BO, Rhodes KP. Toward more rational nerve conduction interpretations: the effect of height. *Muscle and Nerve*. 1990;13.

17.   Soudmand R, Ward LC, Swift TR. Effect of height on nerve conduction velocity. *Neurology*. 1982;32.

18.   Soodan J., Kumar A. Relationship among Anthropometric Indices & Motor Nerve Conduction Velocity of Radial & Ulnar Nerves in Aerobic Trained

Athletes. *J Exerc Sci Physiother*. 2012;8(1).

19. Biewener A a. Biomechanical consequences of scaling. *J Exp Biol*. 2005;208(Pt 9).

20. More HL, Hutchinson JR, Collins DF, Weber DJ, Aung SKH, Donelan JM. Scaling of sensorimotor control in terrestrial mammals. *Proc Biol Sci*. 2010;277(1700).

21. Milgrom C, Shlamkovitch N, Finestone A, et al. Risk factors for lateral ankle sprain: a prospective study among military recruits. *Foot Ankle*. 1991;12(1).

22. Han K-J, Kim Y-K, Lim S-K, Park J-Y, Oh K-S. The effect of physical characteristics and field position on the shoulder and elbow injuries of 490 baseball players: confirmation of diagnosis by magnetic resonance imaging. *Clin J Sport Med*. 2009;19(4).

23. Zwerver J, Bredeweg SW, van den Akker-Scheek I. Prevalence of Jumper's Knee Among Nonelite Athletes From Different Sports: A Cross-Sectional Survey. *Am J Sports Med*. 2011;39(9).

24. Trimpou P, Landin-Wilhelmsen K, Odén a, Rosengren a, Wilhelmsen L. Male risk factors for hip fracture-a 30-year follow-up study in 7,495 men. *Osteoporos Int*. 2010;21(3).

25. Sobti A, Cooper C, Inskip H, Searle S, Coggon D. Occupational physical activity and long-term risk of musculoskeletal symptoms: a national survey of post office pensioners. *Am J Ind Med*. 1997;32(1).

26. Dehner C, Schick S, Arand M, Elbel M, Hell W, Kramer M. Influence of anthropometry on the kinematics of the cervical spine and the risk of injury in sled tests in female volunteers. *Accid Anal Prev*. 2008.

27. Roquelaure Y, Bodin J, Ha C, et al. Incidence and risk factors for thoracic spine pain in the working population: the French Pays de la Loire study.

Arthritis Care Res (Hoboken). 2014;66(11).

28. Wahlström J, Burström L, Nilsson T, Järvholm B. Risk Factors for Hospitalization Due to Lumbar Disc Disease. *Spine (Phila Pa 1976)*. 2012;37(15).

29. Milanese S, Grimmer K. School furniture and the user population: an anthropometric perspective. *Ergonomics*. 2004;47(4).

30. Kuh DJ, Coggan D, Mann S, Cooper C, Yusuf E. Height, occupation and back pain in a national prospective study. *Br J Rheumatol*. 1993;32.

31. McKay GD, Goldie P a, Payne WR, Oakes BW. Ankle injuries in basketball: injury rate and risk factors. *Br J Sports Med*. 2001;35(2).

32. Venturelli M, Schena F, Zanolla L, Bishop D. Injury risk factors in young soccer players detected by a multivariate survival model. *J Sci Med Sport*. 2011;14(4).

33. Wright KJ, Crée C De. The Influence of Somatotype, Strength and Flexibility on Injury Occurrence among Female Competitive Olympic Style Gymnasts. A Pilot Study. *Jounral Phys Ther Sci*. 1998.

34. Jokinen H, Pulkkinen P, Korpelainen J, et al. Risk factors for cervical and trochanteric hip fractures in elderly women: a population-based 10-year follow-up study. *Calcif Tissue Int*. 2010;87(1).

35. McGill SM. *Low Back Disorders: Evidence-Based Prevention and Rehabilitation*. Third Edit. Champaign Illinois: Human Kinetics Publishers; 2002.

36. Scannell JP, McGill SM. Disc prolapse: evidence of reversal with repeated extension. *Spine (Phila Pa 1976)*. 2009;34(4).

37. Kroeber M, Unglaub F, Guehring T, et al. Effects of controlled dynamic disc distraction on degenerated

intervertebral discs: an in vivo study on the rabbit lumbar spine model. *Spine (Phila Pa 1976)*. 2005;30(2).

38.   Adams MA. THE BIOMECHANICS OF BACK PAIN. *Acupunct Med J Br Med Acupunct Soc*. 2003;22(1).

39.   Janda V. Die muskularen hauptsyndrome bei vertebragen en beschwerden, theroetische fortschritte und pracktishe erfahrungen der manuellen medizin. *Int Congr FIMM*. 1979.

40.   Lucett SC. *NASM Essentials of Corrective Exercise Training*.; 2013.

41.   Holtzman S, Beggs RT. Yoga for chronic low back pain: a meta-analysis of randomized controlled trials. *Pain Res Manag*. 2013;18(5).

42.   Cramer H, Lauche R, Haller H, Dobos G. A systematic review and meta-analysis of yoga for low back pain. *Clin J Pain*. 2013;29(5).

43.   Banth S, Ardebil MD. Effectiveness of mindfulness meditation on pain and quality of life of patients with chronic low back pain. *Int J Yoga*. 2015;8(2).

44.   DC C, KJ S, BH B, et al. Effect of mindfulness-based stress reduction vs cognitive behavioral therapy or usual care on back pain and functional limitations in adults with chronic low back pain: A randomized clinical trial. *JAMA*. 2016;315(12).

45.   Rainville J, Hartigan C, Martinez E, Limke J, Jouve C, Finno M. Exercise as a treatment for chronic low back pain. *Spine J*. 2004;4(1).

46.   Naugle KM, Fillingim RB, Riley JL. A meta-analytic review of the hypoalgesic effects of exercise. *J Pain*. 2012;13(12).

47.   Fussa J, Steinlea J, Bindilac L, et al. A runner's high depends on cannabinoid receptors in mice. In:

Proceedings of the National Academy of Sciences. ; 2015.

48.   Rayman MP, Pattison DJ. Dietary manipulation in musculoskeletal conditions. *Best Pract Res Clin Rheumatol.* 2008;22(3).

49.   Marx K. Capital: Volume One. *Karl Marx Sel Writings.* 1977;1; 1(1999).

50.   T-SHIRTS UNRAVELLED. Threadbase.

51.   Cohen A. *The Tall Book: A Celebration of Life from on High.* Bloomsbury USA; 2009.

52.   Justice M of. *Motor Vehicle Safety Regulations.* Canada; 2015.

53.   Boer ER, Bruin J de, Abbink D de, Ward NJ de, Manser M de. Are Drivers with Small Feet or Long Legs at Greater Risk of Rear end Collisions. In: *Proceedings of the Human Factors and Ergonomics Society Annual Meeting.* ; 2006.

54.   Yoganandan N, Baisden JL, Maiman DJ, Pintar FA. Type II odontoid fracture from frontal impact: case report and biomechanical mechanism of injury. *J Neurosurg Spine.* 2005;2(4).

55.   Sochor MR, Faust DP, Wang SC, Schneider LW. Knee , Thigh and Hip Injury Patterns for Drivers and Right Front Passengers in Frontal Impacts Reprinted From⬚: Biomechanics. *Injury.* 2003;(724).

56.   Chong M, Sochor M, Ipaktchi K, Brede C, Poster C, Wang S. The interaction of "occupant factors" on the lower extremity fractures in frontal collision of motor vehicle crashes based on a level I trauma center. *J Trauma.* 2007;62(3).

57.   Untaroiu C, Kerrigan J, Kam C, et al. Correlation of strain and loads measured in the long bones with observed kinematics of the lower limb during vehicle-

pedestrian impacts. *Stapp Car Crash J.* 2007;51(October).

58.   Causse J, Wang X, Denninger L. An experimental investigation on the requirement of roof height and sill width for car ingress and egress. *Ergonomics.* 2012;(October 2014).

59.   WARD JS, KIRKa NS. The Relation between Some Anthropometric Dimensions and Preferred Working Surface Heights in the Kitchen. *Ergonomics.* 1970.

60.   Martin JC, Spirduso WW. Determinants of maximal cycling power: Crank length, pedaling rate and pedal speed. *Eur J Appl Physiol.* 2001;84(5).

61.   Chang S-K, Drury CG. Task demands and human capabilities in door use. *Appl Ergon.* 2007;38(3).

62.   SAKAKIBARA R, TSUNOYAMA K, HOSOI H, et al. Influence of Body Position on Defecation in Humans. *Low Urin Tract Symptoms.* 2010.

63.   Sikirov D. Comparison of straining during defecation in three positions: Results and implications for human health. *Dig Dis Sci.* 2003;48(7).

64.   Services M. US army Standards of Medical Fitness. 2007.

65.   Nasa. Austronaut Requirements.

66.   Lai C-Q. How much of human height is genetic and how much is due to nutrition? *Sci Am.* 2006.

67.   Wood AR. Defining the role of common variation in the genomic and biological architecture of adult human height. *Nat Genet.* 2014;46(11).

68.   Kabat GC, Kim MY, Hollenbeck AR, Rohan TE. Attained height , sex , and risk of cancer at different anatomic sites in the NIH-AARP Diet and Health Study. 2014.

69.   Grasgruber P, Cacek J, Kalina T, Sebera M. The role of

nutrition and genetics as key determinants of the positive height trend. *Econ Hum Biol*. 2014;15.

70.   Schönbeck Y, Talma H, van Dommelen P, et al. The world's tallest nation has stopped growing taller: the height of Dutch children from 1955 to 2009. *Pediatr Res*. 2013;73(3).

71.   Hoecker JL. What's the best way to predict a child's height? Mayo Clinic.

72.   Kanaka G, Kitsiou S, Mavrou A, et al. Tall stature, insulin resistance, and disturbed behavior in a girl with the triple X syndrome harboring three SHOX genes: offspring of a father with mosaic Klinefelter syndrome but with two maternal X chromosomes. *Horm Res*. 2004.

73.   Keizer-schrama SMPFDEM. Sex Steroid Treatment of Constitutionally Tall Stature *. *Endocr Rev*. 1998;19(5).

74.   de Waal WJ, Greyn-Fokker MH, Stijnen T, et al. Accuracy of final height prediction and effect of growth-reductive therapy in 362 constitutionally tall children. *J Clin Endocrinol Metab*. 1996;81(3).

75.   Benyi E, Kieler H, Linder M, et al. Risks of malignant and non-malignant tumours in tall women treated with high-dose oestrogen during adolescence. *Horm Res Paediatr*. 2014.

76.   Hendriks a EJ, Drop SLS, Laven JSE, Boot a M. Fertility of tall girls treated with high-dose estrogen, a dose-response relationship. *J Clin Endocrinol Metab*. 2012;97(9).

77.   Hindmarsh P, Pringle P, Di Silvio L, Brook C. A preliminary report on the role of somatostatin analogue (SMS 201-995) in the management of children with tall stature. *Clin Endocrinol (Oxf)*. 1990.

78. Sheridan C. Gene therapy finds its niche. *Nat Biotechnol*. 2011;29(2).

79. Kiuru M, Crystal RG. Progress and prospects: gene therapy for performance and appearance enhancement. *Gene Ther*. 2008;15(5).

80. Rayner JA, Pyett P, Astbury J. The medicalisation of "tall" girls: A discourse analysis of medical literature on the use of synthetic oestrogen to reduce female height. *Soc Sci Med*. 2010;71(6).

81. Bruinsma FJ, Venn AJ, Patton GC, et al. Concern about tall stature during adolescence and depression in later life. *J Affect Disord*. 2006;91(2-3).

82. MacMullen J. Union intends to provide cardiac screening for retired NBA players. ESPN.

83. Nuesch E, Dale C, Palmer TM, et al. Adult height, coronary heart disease and stroke: a multi-locus Mendelian randomization meta-analysis. *Int J Epidemiol*. 2015.

84. Paajanen T a, Oksala NKJ, Kuukasjärvi P, Karhunen PJ. Short stature is associated with coronary heart disease: a systematic review of the literature and a meta-analysis. *Eur Heart J*. 2010;31(14).

85. Tan SY, Myers J, Froelicher VF. Relationship Between Stature and the Prevalence of Atrial Fibrillation and Cardiovascular Mortality. *Am Hear Assoc*. 2006.

86. Aristotle. On Longevity and Shortness of Life. In: *Great Books of the Western World*. Vol 7. ; 1990:710-713.

87. Dobson GP. On being the right size: Heart design, mitochondrial efficiency and lifespan potential. *Clin Exp Pharmacol Physiol*. 2003;30(8).

88. Rubner M. Das Problem det Lebensdaur und seiner beziehunger zum Wachstum und Ernarnhung. 1908.

89.   Dieckmann K-P, Hartmann JT, Classen J, Lüdde R, Diederichs M, Pichlmeier U. Tallness is associated with risk of testicular cancer: evidence for the nutrition hypothesis. *Br J Cancer*. 2008;99(9).

90.   Wirén S, Häggström C, Ulmer H, et al. Pooled cohort study on height and risk of cancer and cancer death. *Cancer Causes Control*. 2014;25(2).

91.   Nagy JD, Victor EM, Cropper JH. Why don't all whales have cancer? A novel hypothesis resolving Peto's paradox. *Integr Comp Biol*. 2007;47(2).

92.   Peto R, Roe FJ, Lee PN, Levy L, Clack J. Cancer and ageing in mice and men. *Br J Cancer*. 1975;32(4).

93.   Maciak S, Michalak P. Cell size and cancer: a new solution to Peto's paradox? *Evol Appl*. 2015;8(1).

94.   Katzourakis A, Magiorkinis G, Lim AG, Gupta S, Belshaw R, Gifford R. Larger mammalian body size leads to lower retroviral activity. *PLoS Pathog*. 2014;10(7).

95.   LM A, AF C, A C, et al. POtential mechanisms for cancer resistance in elephants and comparative cellular response to dna damage in humans. *JAMA*. 2015.

96.   Rosenberg MA, Patton KK, Sotoodehnia N, et al. The impact of height on the risk of atrial fibrillation: the Cardiovascular Health Study. *Eur Hear J*. 2012;33(21).

97.   Hanna IR, Heeke B, Bush H, et al. The Relationship Between Stature and the Prevalence of Atrial Fibrillation in Patients With Left Ventricular Dysfunction. *J Am Coll Cardiol*. 2006;47.

98.   Reiffel JA. Atrial fibrillation and stroke: epidemiology. *Am J Med*. 2014;127(4).

99.   Samaras TT, Bartke A, Rollo CD. *Human Body Size and the Laws of Scaling: Physiological, Performance,*

Growth, Longevity and Ecological Ramifications. Vol 16.; 2007.

100.   Samaras TT. Evidence from Eight Different Types of Studies Showing that Smaller Body Size is Related to Greater Longevity. *J Sci Res Reports*. 2014;3(16).

101.   Herskind AM, McGue M, Holm N V, Sørensen TI, Harvald B, Vaupel JW. The heritability of human longevity: a population-based study of 2872 Danish twin pairs born 1870-1900. *Hum Genet*. 1996;97(3).

102.   Dato S, Crocco P, D'Aquila P, et al. Exploring the role of genetic variability and lifestyle in oxidative stress response for healthy aging and longevity. *Int J Mol Sci*. 2013;14(8).

103.   BBeliveau R, Gingras D. *Foods That Fight Cancer: Preventing Cancer through Diet.*; 2003.

104.   Pollan M. *In Defense of Food: An Eater's Manifesto.*; 2007.

105.   Lakoff G, Johnson M. Metaphors We Live By. *Prod Real essays Read Soc Interact*. 1997.

106.   Patzer G. *The Power and Paradox of Physical Attractiveness.*; 2006.

107.   Judge T a, Cable DM. The effect of physical height on workplace success and income: preliminary test of a theoretical model. *J Appl Psychol*. 2004;89(3).

108.   Dalgaard C-J, Strulik H. A physiological foundation for the nutrition-based efficiency wage model. *Oxf Econ Pap*. 2011;63(2).

109.   Schumacher A. On the significance of stature in human society. *J Hum Evol*. 1982;11(8).

110.   Case A, Paxson C. Stature and Status: Height, Ability, and Labor Market Outcomes. *J Polit Econ*. 2008;116(3).

111. Heineck G. Too tall to be smart? The relationship between height and cognitive abilities. *Econ Lett.* 2009;105(1).

112. Persico N, Postlewaite A, Silverman D. The Effect of Adolescent Experience on Labor Market Outcomes: The Case of Height. *J Polit Econ.* 2004;112(5).

113. Rietveld CA, Hessels J, van der Zwan P. The stature of the self-employed and its relation with earnings and satisfaction. *Econ Hum Biol.* 2015;17.

114. Mueller U, Mazur a. Evidence of unconstrained directional selection for male tallness. *Behav Ecol Sociobiol.* 2001;50(4).

115. TORRE PSS. LARGER THAN REAL LIFE. *Sport Illus.* 2011;(1).

116. Walker B. *Tall Tales: The Great Talisman of Height.*; 2014.

117. Feldman S. The presentation of shortness in everyday life—height and heightism in American society: Toward a sociology of stature Paper. *Am Sociol Assoc.* 1971.

118. Cohen S. *H.R.4490 - SEAT Act of 2016.*; 2016.

119. Finlay Travis K. (Winston-Salem NCUJGA (Rural HSCUVPJ (Winston-SNCU. Method and Apparatus for Adjusting the Spacing of Vehicle Seats Based on the Size of the Seat Occupant. 2015;(20150145300).

120. Riley BB. We're Cramped as Hell, and we Won't Take it Anymore — Plotting a Class Action Disability Claim on Behalf of the Very Tall Against Air Carriers for a Failure to Accomodate. 2013.

121. Disabilities. Wolrd Health Organization.

122. Mankiw G, Weinzierl M. The Optimal Taxation of Height: A Case Study of Utilitarian Income Redistribution. *Am Econ J Econ Policy.* 2010;2(1).

123.   Coyne D. Grave decision ahead for Ballina council. Echo Netdaily.

124.   Fox T, Fimeche C. Global food: Waste not, want not. *Inst Mech Eng*. 2013.

125.   Seri. Overconsumption? Our use of the world's natural resources. *Sustain Eur Res Inst*. 2009.

126.   Stulp G, Buunk AP, Kurzban R, Verhulst S. The height of choosiness: Mutual mate choice for stature results in suboptimal pair formation for both sexes. *Anim Behav*. 2013;86(1).

127.   Weitzman A, Conley D. *From Assortative to Ashortative Coupling: Men's Height, Height Heterogamy, and Relationship Dynamics in the United States*.; 2014.

128.   Nettle D. Women's height, reproductive success and the evolution of sexual dimorphism in modern humans. *Proc Biol Sci*. 2002;269(1503).

129.   Blaker NM, Rompa I, Dessing IH, Vriend AF, Herschberg C, Van Vugt M. The height leadership advantage in men and women: Testing evolutionary psychology predictions about the perceptions of tall leaders. *Gr Process Intergr Relations*. 2013;16(1).

130.   Alexander K.C. Leung, W Lane M. Robson N. Evaluating tall children. *Can Fam Physician*. 1995.

131.   Farman TC. Should women fear being too tall? A study examining the experiences of very tall women. *ProQuest Diss Theses*. 2010.

132.   Sohn K. Does a taller husband make his wife happier? *Pers Individ Dif*. 2016;91.

133.   Firmin MW, Hoffman SJ, Firmin RL, Lee AD, Vorobyov Y. Tall College Women's Social Dynamics Relating to Height. *Qual Res Psychol*. 2012;9(3).

134.   Meisenberg G. The reproduction of intelligence.

Intelligence. 2010;38(2).

About the Author

Sam Lochner received his PhD in mechanical engineering from the University of Waterloo in 2013. His work and research relates to mass customization and biomechanics. At 6'7", he has experienced both the pros and cons of being tall. In particular, it was central in both reaching the provincial volleyball level but then becoming a chronic back pain suffer. Yet by drawing on his engineering aptitude, he was able to recover. This, and other experiences related to his height, inspired him to write this book.

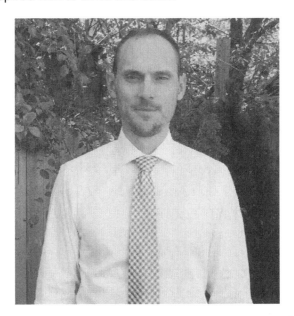

25377301R00105

Printed in Great Britain
by Amazon